Healthy Diet Plan: 2 Manuscripts

ANTI INFLAMMATORY RECIPES

Delicious Healthy Foods to Make at Home

And

A Leptin Mediterranean Diet

Over 50 Enticing Recipes To Energise Your Day

By: Emily Simmons

© Copyright 2019 - by Emily Simmons All rights reserved.

The content contained within this book may not be reproduced, duplicated or transmitted without direct written permission from the author or the publisher.

Under no circumstances will any blame or legal responsibility be held against the publisher, or author, for any damages, reparation, or monetary loss due to the information contained within this book, either directly or indirectly.

Legal Notice:

This book is copyright protected. It is only for personal use. You cannot amend, distribute, sell, use, quote or paraphrase any part, or the content within this book, without the consent of the author or publisher.

Disclaimer Notice:

Please note the information contained within this document is for educational and entertainment purposes only. All effort has been executed to present accurate, up to date, reliable, complete information. No warranties of any kind are declared or implied. Readers acknowledge that the author is not engaging in the rendering of legal, financial, medical or professional advice. The content within this book has been derived from various sources. Please consult a licensed professional before attempting any techniques outlined in this book.

By reading this document, the reader agrees that under no circumstances is the author responsible for any losses, direct or indirect, that are incurred as a result of the use of information contained within this document, including, but not limited to, errors, omissions, or inaccuracies.

Table of Contents

Book 1: Anti Inflammatory Recipes-11

Introduction-12

BREAKFASTS-15

Tropical Smoothie-17

Passion Fruit and Blueberry Smoothie-18

Fruit and Yogurt Meal in a Glass-20

Pomegranate Jewel Bowls with Peaches and Yoghurt-22

Spicy Gingerbread Oatmeal-24

Creamy Nutty Oatmeal Porridge-26

Poached Eggs with Swiss Chard-27

Sweet Potato Frittata with Tomato Relish-30

Strawberry Drinking Yogurt-32

For breakfast or even for when you're craving a milkshake,you're sure to love this yummy pink treat.-32

Cashew-Butter Toast-33

Vegetable Breakfast Frittata-34

Mushroom Omelets with Thyme-36

SOUPS-38

French Vegetable Soup-39

Barley and White Bean Soup-40

Spicy Lentil and Vegetable Soup-43

Golden Yellow Soup-45

Butternut and Sweet Potato Soup with Ginger-47

Pumpkin Soup with Pine Nuts-49

Zucchini Soup-51

Lentil Soup-52

SALADS-55

Spinach Salad with Oranges and Walnuts-56

Modern Cobb Salad-57

Two Bean Salad-58

Chopped Salad with Avocado Dressing-59

Japanese Inspired Salad-60

Spring Greens and Pineapple Salad-61

Crisp Clean Coleslaw-64

DINNERS-66

Baked Chicken-67

Shrimp Pasta-69

Thai Red Curry-70

Curried Potatoes in Tomato Sauce with Eggs-73

Turkey Bolognese-75

Roasted Chicken with Lemon, Baby Potatoes, and Broccoli-77

Cinnamon Baked Lamb with Butternut Squash-79

Chicken and Mushroom Pilaf-81

Salmon and Zucchini with Lemon and Herbs-83

Basic Stir-Fry-85

Pan-Fried Salmon on Rocket Salad-87

Nonna's Stew-89

SWEET TREATS-91

Strawberry Banana Frozen Yogurt-91

Oatmeal Cashew Cookies-93

Honey-Ginger Syrupy Baked Pears-95

Crustless Apple and Cranberry Pie-97

Raisin and Spice Cookies-99

Oat Cookies-102

Minty Berry Sorbet-104

Conclusion-106

Introduction-110

LEPTIN-MEDITERRANEAN HEALTHY BREAKFAST RECIPES-115

Mediterranean Ham and Egg Cups-115

Mediterranean Chicken Quiche-119

Mediterranean Beef Frittata-122

Mediterranean Egg Muffins-126

Mediterranean Vegetable Cakes-128

Mediterranean Breakfast Sandwiches-131

Potato Hash with Chickpea-134

Banana Nut Oatmeal-137

Melamen-139

Mediterranean Chicken Stir-Fry-141

LEPTIN MEDITERRANEAN HEALTHY LUNCH RECIPES-144

Mediterranean Salmon Salad-144

Spinach Salad with Chicken, Avocado, and Goat Cheese-147

Greek Chicken Souvlaki Salad-152

Baked Chicken Stuffed with Pesto and Cheese-155

Marsala Chicken and Mushroom Casserole-157

Low-Carb Tuscan Soup-161

Crockpot Low -Carb Spicy Chicken Soup-163

Low-Carb Avgolemono (Greek Chicken, Lemon & Egg Soup)- 165

Cream of Roasted Cauliflower Soup, with Cumin, Paprika, and Fresh Dill-167

LEPTIN MEDITERRANEAN HEALTHY DINNER RECIPES-171

Mediterranean Shrimp over Spinach-171

Mediterranean Low-Carb "Cauliflower Risotto"- 174

Mediterranean Baked Fish, with Tomato- Onion- Garlic Sauce-176

Shrimp Saganaki-178

Grilled Shrimp Salad with Feta, Tomato, and Watermelon-180

Orecchiette with Mussels & Mint-183

Greek-Style Shrimp Salad-185

Halibut and Mussel Stew with Fennel, Peppers, and Saffron-187

Tilapia Feta Florentine-191

A richly satisfying bake, full of nutritious goodness. 191

Bake it in oven for 20 to 25 minutes, or until the fish is flaky and cooked through. Gyro Salad-192

LEPTIN MEDITERRANEAN HEALTHY SOUP RECIPES-195

Cabbage Soup with Kielbasa-195

Chilled Red Pepper Soup with Sautéed Shrimp-198

Grilled Watermelon Gazpacho with Lime Cream-200

White Gazpacho with Grapes and Toasted Almonds-202

Mediterranean Kale & White Bean Soup with Sausage-204

Moroccan Vegetable Ragoût-206

Cucumber-Yogurt Soup with Avocado-208

Roasted Red Pepper & Tomato Gazpacho-211

Mediterranean Roasted Vegetable Soup-215

LEPTIN MEDITERRANEAN HEALTHY SALAD RECIPES-218

Mediterranean Cucumber & Tomato Salad-218

Feta Salad with Pomegranate Dressing-220

Fig & Mozzarella salad-**223**

Shredded Romaine and Cucumber Salad with Yogurt Dressing-**225**

Brooklyn Grange Salad with Pickled Eggs and Idiazabal-**229**

Poached Quince Salad-**232**

Farro Salad with Marinated Artichokes, Watercress, and Feta-**234**

Grilled Eggplant Salad with Feta, Pine Nuts & Garlicky Yogurt Dressing-**237**

Tomato Salad with Feta, Olives & Mint-**239**

Conclusion-**241**

ANTI INFLAMMATORY RECIPES

Delicious Healthy Foods to Make at Home

By: Emily Simmons

Introduction

Welcome, and congratulations on your purchase of a recipe book that I hope you'll use over and over in the coming days. This book aims to help you nourish your body with foods that will fight inflammation, by the use of nature's own medicines- fresh unprocessed foods, herbs, and spices.

So, who needs this book? Anyone who may be suffering from a chronic disease, as well as anyone who may wish to avoid such diseases. The book will introduce you to easily obtainable foods that you should incorporate into your diet, and will then feature them in easy to prepare, delicious recipes for you to make at home, without having to spend hours in the kitchen.

First though, we need to look at what inflammation in the body is, what causes it, and why it's not always a good thing. Since the 1980's, researchers have discovered a relationship between certain foods and certain chronic (long-term) diseases such as cancer, diabetes, arthritis, and others. They have discovered that certain foods cause inflammation in our bodies, and others calm it.

The body is actually made to use inflammation in a good way, such as to cause swelling around a wound to help seal it off, or to protect the wound from infection. However, when inflammation gets out of control, it becomes a bad thing. Sometimes the inflammatory response in the body can be so extreme that it contributes to the development of diseases such as cancer, diabetes, arthritis, and heart disease. This happens when the immune system's inflammatory response over-reacts, and instead of only attacking viruses and bacteria, or clearing out damaged cells, it starts to attack healthy cells as well.

Controlling what we eat goes a long way to controlling how our immune system will respond to threats. Different people respond differently to different foods. For example, some people feel bloated and uncomfortable after eating bread or dairy products, yet others tolerate these foodstuffs well. Some foods, however, are known to cause problems for a lot of people, and these are the ones to start eliminating from your diet first. Don't worry, though, we won't be just taking foods away from you, but we'll be making replacements with other easily tolerated, scrumptious eats. An easy way to tell what foods are best to avoid is by keeping in mind that the further removed from its natural state a product is, the more likely it is to cause inflammation in the body. (e.g. apple pie.) The closer foods are to the way they were created, the less likely they are to cause harm. (e.g. an apple.) Because of this, some of the recipes in this book are not so much recipes, as ideas for combining simple, fresh foods in a new way, sometimes without even having to cook. What could be easier than that? The way that foods are prepared also makes a difference to their nutritional value and to whether or not they will cause an inflammatory response. Deep frying your fish, for example, can change what was a health giving food into one that may cause harm. Baking it with a sprinkle of olive oil and lemon juice and a few herbs, however, keeps it tasty and retains all its nutritional value.

An interesting new finding is the role that spices and herbs can play in fighting inflammation in our bodies. Some common herbs and spices that you probably already have in your kitchen are on the list, and many have been included in the recipes which follow.

You'll want to avoid too many foods that contain omega 6's. Not because they are bad in themselves, but because our ratio of omega 3's to omega 6's should be about 1:1. Since nowadays we tend to have far more omega 3's than 6's in our diets, contributing to inflammation, we need to reduce the amount of omega 6's we consume.

BREAKFASTS

We all know that breakfast is a super-important meal, but how many of us have spare time in the morning? This chapter aims to give you ideas and recipes that are quick and easy to prepare, and that give you a boost of nutrients to get your day off to a good start. Remember, food is your body's fuel, so just as you wouldn't start a trip by filling your car with inferior quality fuel, neither should you start off your day by filling your body with inferior food.

If you stock up on fresh or frozen fruit, natural Greek yoghurt, nuts and seeds, and some eggs, you'll never be short of a quick and simple breakfast.

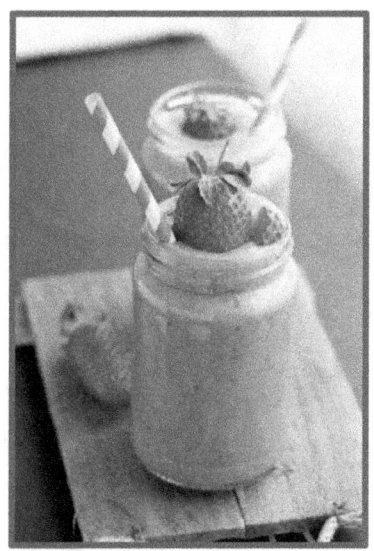

Tropical Smoothie

Making a smoothie in the morning is a really fast and easy way to pack in a lot of nutrients and hydrating liquid without having to make a huge meal.

INGREDIENTS:

½ cup coconut milk

½ cup almond milk

1 ripe banana, peeled and sliced

½ teaspoon ground cinnamon

1 tablespoon flax seeds, ground

INSTRUCTIONS:

Combine the coconut milk, almond milk, banana, cinnamon, and ground flax seeds in a blender. Blend until smooth. Pour into a tall glass and serve.

Serves 1

Passion Fruit and Blueberry Smoothie

Blueberries are among the most nutrient dense berries, and are considered a superfood. Passion fruits are rich in vitamin C. So together, they make for a really good way to begin the morning.

INGREDIENTS:

2 passion fruits, seeds scooped out into blender

1 ripe banana, peeled and sliced

1 cup fresh blueberries

2 tablespoons fresh lemon juice

1 cup plain low-fat Greek yogurt, or dairy-free milk such as almond

2 teaspoons honey

1 teaspoon cinnamon

INSTRUCTIONS:

Put the passion fruit, banana, blueberries, and lemon juice in a blender and blend together until smooth.

Add the yogurt, honey, and cinnamon and blend again.

Pour into glasses and serve immediately.

Serves 2-3

Fruit and Yogurt Meal in a Glass

Combine chunks of whatever fruit you have on hand, and make a superbly healthy breakfast in just a few minutes. Flax seeds are very high in omega 3's, and should be ground to make all the micronutrients easy to absorb.

INGREDIENTS:

1 cup plain low- fat yoghurt

A few drops of vanilla extract

½ cup fruit such as blueberries, raspberries, bananas, strawberries, or peaches, chopped into small dice

1 tablespoon flax seeds, ground

2 tablespoons walnuts, chopped

1 teaspoon honey, to serve

INSTRUCTIONS:

Mix the yoghurt and vanilla, and place half the yoghurt into a tall parfait glass. Top with half of the fruit, and sprinkle with half of the ground flax and the walnuts. Layer the remaining yoghurt on top, then the remaining fruit, nuts and seeds. Drizzle with the honey. Serve at once.

Serves 1

Pomegranate Jewel Bowls with Peaches and Yoghurt

Pomegranates are beautiful, and they've been found to have three times the antioxidants as red wine or green tea. They have potent anti-inflammatory effects, especially in diabetics.

INGREDIENTS:

1 cup fresh peaches, sliced

1/2 cup plain low-fat Greek yogurt

1 teaspoon honey

1 tablespoon flax seeds, ground

2 tablespoons fresh pomegranate seeds

Handful of almonds, chopped

INSTRUCTIONS:

Arrange the peach slices in a bowl and top with the yogurt; then drizzle with the honey.

Sprinkle with the flax seeds, pomegranate seeds, and almonds.

Serves 1

Spicy Gingerbread Oatmeal

This is a warm, comforting breakfast that will warm your tummy on those icy winter mornings. It's full of spices known for their anti-inflammatory effects.

INGREDIENTS:

1 cup steel cut oats

4 cups water

Pinch of salt

1 teaspoons ground cinnamon

½ teaspoon ground ginger

Maple syrup to taste

INSTRUCTIONS:

Put the oats, water, and salt in a saucepan and bring to the boil. Reduce the heat and simmer gently for about 15 minutes, stirring now and then. Add the spices and stir to mix. Serve the porridge hot, drizzled with maple syrup. Serve with a little milk if you like.

Serves 4

Creamy Nutty Oatmeal Porridge

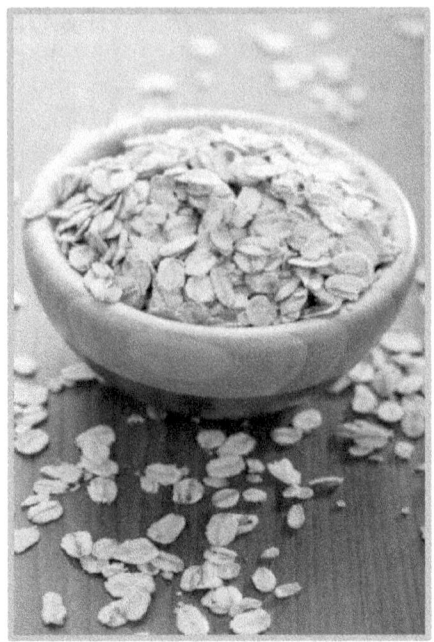

Another version of oatmeal porridge that's quick to make and provides a filling breakfast to set you up for a busy day.

INGREDIENTS:

4 cups water

1 cup steel-cut oats

Pinch of salt

1 tablespoon flax seeds, ground

¼ cup mixed raw nuts, such as cashews, almonds, or walnuts, chopped

2 tablespoons almond milk

1 teaspoon honey, or ½ teaspoon stevia

INSTRUCTIONS:

In a medium sized saucepan bring the water and oats to the boil, with a big pinch of salt. Reduce the heat to low, and simmer for about 15 minutes. Stir in the ground flax, nuts, and milk. Drizzle honey over the top. Serve hot.

Serves 1

Poached Eggs with Swiss Chard

Sometimes one just feels like a savory breakfast. Eggs are a great way to start off the day, because they're full of protein and other nutrients such as omega 3's and vitamin D. A breakfast of eggs can keep you fuller for longer and eliminate the need for a lot of snacking through the morning. An added benefit is that, for most people, eggs are anti-inflammatory. In fact, people who eat a steady breakfast of eggs, fresh fruit, and a cup of coffee can reduce their inflammation markers by up to 20 percent. It's perfectly safe to eat up to four eggs a week.

INGREDIENTS:

2 eggs

2 slices oat bread

2 teaspoons extra-virgin olive oil

1 bunch of Swiss chard, well washed, shredded

2 tablespoons chopped fresh parsley

Sea salt and freshly ground pepper to taste

INSTRUCTIONS:

Using a small frying pan, lightly stir-fry the Swiss chard in the oil until wilted and most of the water has evaporated. Season with salt and pepper.

For the eggs, bring 2 cups of water, with a teaspoon of vinegar added, to a gentle boil in a shallow pan. Break one egg into a small bowl, lower the bowl almost to the water, and tip the egg into the water. Do the same with the second egg.

Use a spoon to nudge the egg whites closer to the yolk, helping to keep the egg whites together. Leave the eggs to poach for about 3 to 4 minutes. Lift the eggs out of the water gently with a slotted spoon.

Toast the bread while the eggs are poaching. To serve, place the toast on a plate, top with Swiss chard, and then with the egg. Serve at once.

Serves 2

Sweet Potato Frittata with Tomato Relish

INGREDIENTS:

1 large sweet potato, peeled and cut into small cubes, boiled till just cooked

4 tablespoon olive oil
2 small onions, peeled and finely chopped

Sea salt and black pepper to taste
4 eggs
handful each of parsley and chives, finely chopped
3 plum tomatoes, peeled and chopped

I red chili, seeded and finely chopped

1 teaspoon agave syrup

INSTRUCTIONS:

To make the relish, heat a tablespoon of oil in a small frying pan. Fry 1 of the onions until softened, then add the tomatoes and chili. Simmer until reduced to a thick saucy relish. Season with agave, salt, and pepper. Set aside.
To make the frittata, first heat the grill (broiler) element.

Using a non-stick omelet pan (one that's ok to use under the grill) add the remaining olive oil. Heat and then add the remaining onion. Season with salt and pepper. Fry until soft, then add the sweet potatoes. Fry until golden. In a bowl, beat the eggs and pour into the skillet over the sweet potatoes. Sprinkle with parsley and chives. Cook on low heat, do not stir, until the eggs start setting. Now put the skillet under the grill to set the top. Be careful not to overcook. Loosen with a spatula and turn out onto a serving dish. Cut in half and serve at once with a dollop of tomato relish on each serving.

Serves 2

Strawberry Drinking Yogurt

For breakfast or even for when you're craving a milkshake, you're sure to love this yummy pink treat.

INGREDIENTS:

1 cup plain low-fat yogurt

½ cup strawberries, fresh or frozen

¼ cup almond milk

1 teaspoon honey or ½ teaspoon stevia

INSTRUCTIONS:

Combine the yogurt, strawberries, almond milk, and honey or stevia in a blender. Blend the ingredients until smooth and pour into a glass. Serve with a straw.

Serves 1

Cashew-Butter Toast

Making your own nut butter couldn't be easier, and it's delicious and filling on toast with honey.

INGREDIENTS:

½ cup unsalted roasted cashews

pinch of salt

2 slices oat bread

1 teaspoon honey

INSTRUCTIONS:

Combine the cashews and the salt in a small food processor bowl and puree until smooth. Toast the bread slices and spread them with the cashew butter. Drizzle the toast with honey.

Serves 1

Vegetable Breakfast Frittata

Yes, you can and should have vegetables for breakfast!

INGREDIENTS:

1 tablespoon extra-virgin olive oil

1 small onion, finely chopped

½ cup fresh vegetables, such as zucchini, spinach, broccoli, and kale, diced

2 eggs, beaten

1 tablespoon goat cheese

Salt and black pepper, to taste

INSTRUCTIONS:

Heat the olive oil in a non-stick frying pan. Sauté the onion in the olive oil for a couple of minutes until it's transparent and soft. Add the remaining vegetables and sauté for a few minutes until softened.

Pour the beaten eggs into the vegetable mixture and cook for a minute until the eggs have set. Don't stir them, just tip the pan as it cooks, lifting the edges of the egg to let the uncooked egg to trickle underneath and cook. When almost done, top with the cheese and season with salt and pepper.

Slide out gently onto a plate.

Serves 1

Mushroom Omelets with Thyme

Mushrooms provide a mineral that's not commonly found in most other fruits or vegetables- selenium. It helps the liver enzymes to function properly, and helps detoxify some cancer-causing compounds in the body. Selenium also prevents inflammation and has been shown to and also decrease tumor growth rates.

INGREDIENTS:

1 tablespoon extra-virgin olive oil

1 small onion, finely chopped

1 clove garlic, finely chopped

1 cup sliced mushrooms

2 eggs, beaten

2 goat cheese, grated or crumbled

2 teaspoons fresh thyme leaves

INSTRUCTIONS:

Heat half of the olive oil in a non-stick frying pan over medium heat. Sauté the onions and garlic until they're translucent and soft. Add the mushrooms and continue to sauté until the mushrooms are soft and the water had evaporated. Set the mushroom mixture aside in a separate bowl and keep warm. Put the rest of the olive oil into the same frying pan you used for the mushrooms, and add the eggs. Don't stir, just tilt the pan and lift the edges of the egg, letting the uncooked egg run underneath. When all the egg has almost set, spoon the mushroom mixture onto one half of the omelet, and top with the cheese and thyme leaves. Season with salt and pepper. Fold the egg over the side with the mushrooms on, and slide out of the pan onto a plate. Serve at once.

Serves 1

SOUPS

Wonderfully aromatic and satisfying, soups are probably the ultimate convenience food. They're also one of the best ways to pack a lot of nutrients into one bowl. The recipes that follow use a lot of pulses, which are high in protein and fiber, and low in fat. They also incorporate many vegetables and recommended anti-inflammatory herbs, such as celery and rosemary. So go ahead and brew a potful!

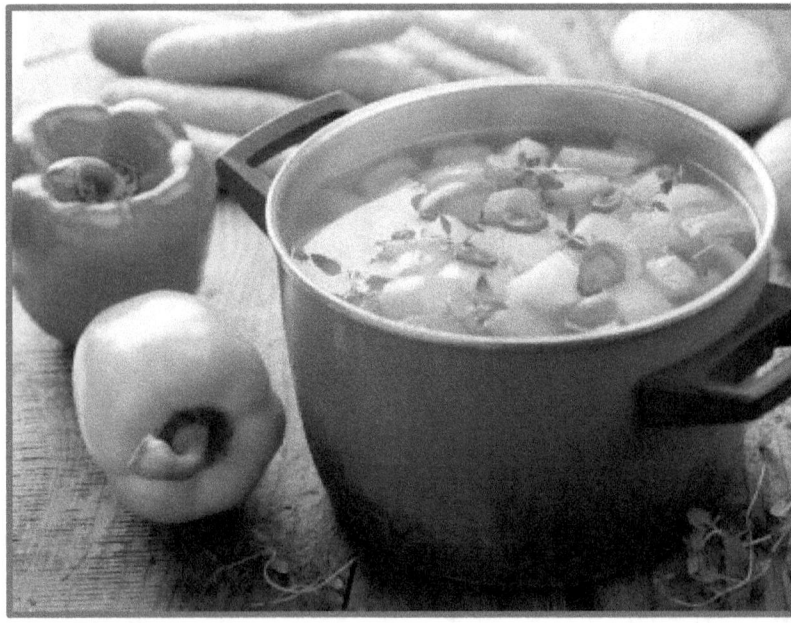

French Vegetable Soup

The addition of basil pesto at the end gives this soup a delightfully fresh flavor.

INGREDIENTS:

2 tablespoons olive oil

1 red onion, finely chopped

2 cloves of garlic, very finely chopped

1 red bell pepper, diced

1 carrot, diced

1 celery stalk, including the leaves, finely chopped

2 cups cabbage, shredded

2 tablespoons fresh oregano

2 cups kale, finely shredded

½ cup lentils

½ cup barley

2 liters vegetable or chicken stock

Handful fresh parsley, finely chopped

Sea salt and freshly ground black pepper, to taste

Basil pesto, to serve

INSTRUCTIONS:

Using a soup pot, heat the oil. Fry the onion, garlic and red pepper till softened. Add carrot, celery, cabbage, oregano, and kale. Stir fry until the vegetables have softened. Add lentils, barley and stock. Bring to a boil, then reduce heat and simmer for about an hour or until the barley and lentils are soft. Add the parsley and some salt and pepper. Serve hot, in warmed bowls, adding a teaspoon of pesto into each bowl.

Serves 8

Barley and White Bean Soup

A substantial and nourishing soup, this is a complete meal in itself. If you don't have fresh herbs, feel free to use dried ones, only be sure to reduce the quantity.

INGREDIENTS:

2 cans cannellini beans (410g each), drained and rinsed

2 tablespoons extra-virgin olive oil

1 onion, diced

2 cloves garlic, finely chopped

2 large carrots, peeled and diced

2 cups chicken or vegetable stock

2 litres water

½ cup barley

2 sticks celery, leaves included, finely shredded

2 tablespoons fresh sage leaves, finely chopped

2 tablespoons fresh rosemary leaves, finely chopped

Sea salt and freshly ground black pepper, to taste

INSTRUCTIONS:

Using a big soup pot, heat the olive oil over medium heat. Sauté the onion, garlic, and carrots for a few minutes until softened. Add the stock, water, barley, and beans to the saucepan. Bring the soup to a boil over high heat.

Lower the heat, add the celery, sage and rosemary, and simmer the soup for about 1 hour, or until the barley is soft. Add more water as needed for the desired thickness. Season the soup to taste with salt and pepper.

Serves 6-8

Spicy Lentil and Vegetable Soup

INGREDIENTS:

2 tablespoons extra-virgin olive oil

1 onion, diced

2 cloves garlic, finely diced

1 large carrot, peeled and diced

1 teaspoon ground coriander seed

1 teaspoon ground cumin seed

½ teaspoon turmeric

2 litres vegetable or chicken stock

500g dried lentils, rinsed

½ cup mustard greens, chopped

Handful of fresh parsley, finely chopped

Juice of 1 lemon

Sea salt and freshly ground black pepper to taste

INSTRUCTIONS:

Using a large soup pot, heat the olive oil and sauté the onions, garlic, and carrot until softened. Add the coriander, cumin, and turmeric, stirring for a few seconds. Add the stock and lentils. Bring to the boil, then turn the heat down and simmer for about 30 minutes until the lentils are no longer firm. Add the mustard greens and parsley and simmer for another few minutes. Season with lemon juice, salt and pepper. Serve hot.

Serves 6-8

Golden Yellow Soup

This soup is a beautiful color, with a slightly sweet flavor. You're sure to make this again and again.

INGREDIENTS:

2 tablespoons extra-virgin olive oil

2 medium onions, peeled and diced

2 carrots, peeled and diced

1 parsnip, peeled and diced

2 litres vegetable or chicken stock

400g dried yellow split peas

1 large sweet potato, peeled and diced

1-2 tablespoons fresh oregano, chopped

Sea salt and freshly ground black pepper to taste

INSTRUCTIONS:

Using a soup pot, heat the oil and sauté the onions, carrots, and parsnips until soft.

Add the stock, split peas, sweet potato, and oregano. Bring the soup to a boil over high heat, and then reduce the heat to simmer for up to 1 hour or until all the vegetables and peas are mushy and the soup is as thick as you want. Season the soup to taste with salt and pepper.

Serves 6

Butternut and Sweet Potato Soup with Ginger

Besides being delicious, ginger is also a powerful anti-inflammatory. Some studies have shown that it's effective at reducing the symptoms of osteoarthritis, a common inflammatory disease. It has also been shown to lower blood sugars and even helps with digestion. In this smooth creamy soup, it combines well with the flavors of butternut and sweet potato.

INGREDIENTS:

2 tablespoons extra-virgin olive oil

1 medium onion, chopped

6 cups vegetable or chicken stock

1 butternut squash, peeled and cubed

1 large sweet potato

3cm piece of fresh ginger, peeled and finely grated

Sea salt to taste

1 tablespoon fresh cream per serving, to serve

INSTRUCTIONS:

Using a soup pot, heat the oil and sauté the onions until they are soft. Add the stock, butternut, sweet potato, and ginger to the pot. Bring to the boil, reduce heat and simmer for about 20 minutes until the vegetables are very soft. Allow the soup to cool for a few minutes before transferring it to a blender or food processor. Blend the soup until it's smooth. Check the seasoning. Serve in bowls with a spoonful of cream in each.

Serves 6

Pumpkin Soup with Pine Nuts

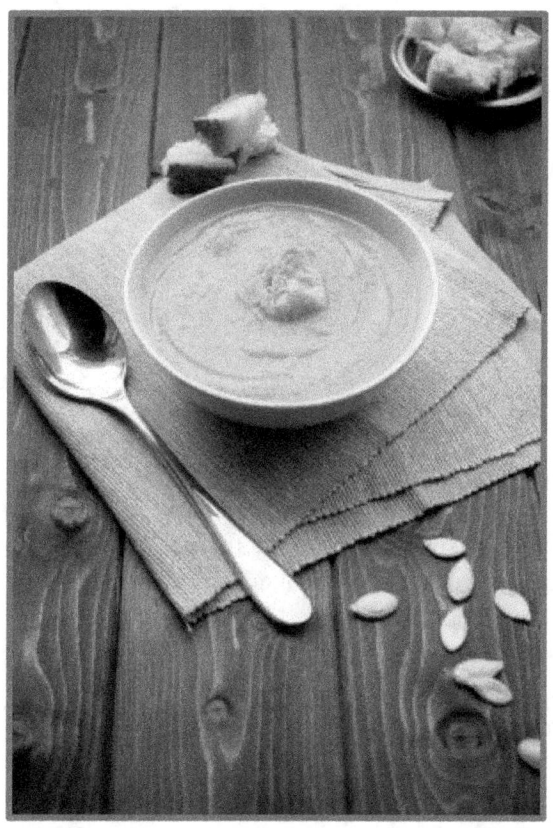

Pine nuts are a good source of vitamin E, zinc, iron, and many other nutrients. Their nutty chewiness is perfect when combined with this smooth, creamy soup, which is ready to eat in about half an hour.

INGREDIENTS:

1 ½ litres chicken or vegetable stock

1 medium pumpkin, seeded, peeled, and chopped

1 large onion, chopped

1 teaspoon ground cinnamon

2 teaspoons honey

pine nuts to serve

INSTRUCTIONS:

Using a soup pot, put the stock into it and bring to the boil. Add the pumpkin, onion, and cinnamon. Turn down the heat and simmer the soup for about 20 minutes until the pumpkin is cooked. Stir in the honey and add salt and pepper if needed. Remove from the heat and allow to cool slightly. Put it in a blender and blend or the soup until it's smooth. Return it to the pot to reheat, then serve in bowls with a sprinkling of pine nuts on top.

Serves 6

Zucchini Soup

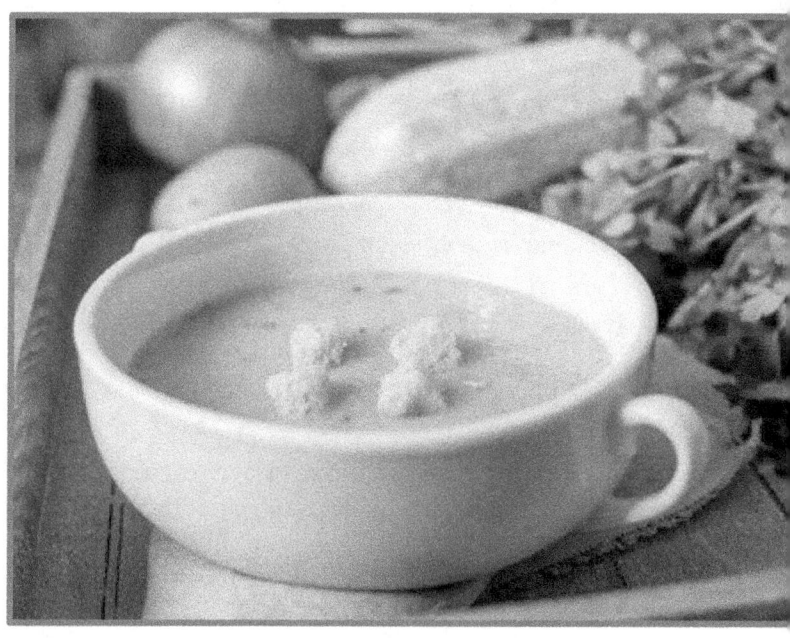

A fresh, summery soup, this is useful as a starter or it can be served as a main course with some chunky whole-wheat bread.

INGREDIENTS:

3 tablespoons extra-virgin olive oil

4 cups zucchini, grated

1 clove garlic, finely chopped

1 onion, chopped

¼ cup fresh parsley

6 cups vegetable or chicken stock

INSTRUCTIONS:

Using a soup pot, heat the olive oil over medium heat. Sauté the zucchini, garlic, and onion until they're soft. Add the parsley and stock. Bring the soup to the boil, then turn the heat down and simmer for 30 minutes. Serve hot.

Serves 8

Lentil Soup

This tasty soup provides lots of anti-inflammatory spices, and is gluten free.

INGREDIENTS:

1 tablespoon coconut oil

2 onions, peeled and finely chopped

3 cloves of garlic, crushed

1 teaspoon turmeric

1 tablespoon fresh ginger, finely grated

1 tsp ground cumin

1 tsp masala

1 teaspoon dried chili

½ tsp ground cinnamon

I large carrot, finely grated

1 cup lentils, rinsed

1 ½ cups vegetable or chicken stock

1 ½ cups coconut milk

INSTRUCTIONS:

Using a soup pot, heat the oil and fry the onion and garlic until softened. Add the turmeric, ginger, cumin, masala, chili, and cinnamon and cook for a few minutes until smelling gorgeous. Add the lentils, stock, and coconut milk. Bring to boil then reduce heat to low and simmer, uncovered, for about half an hour, or until the lentils are mushy and have absorbed most of the liquid. Serve hot.

Serves 4

SALADS

Fresh and crunchy, salads are also so quick and easy to prepare. Try having a salad every day before your main meal to help you get your nutrient quota in for the day.

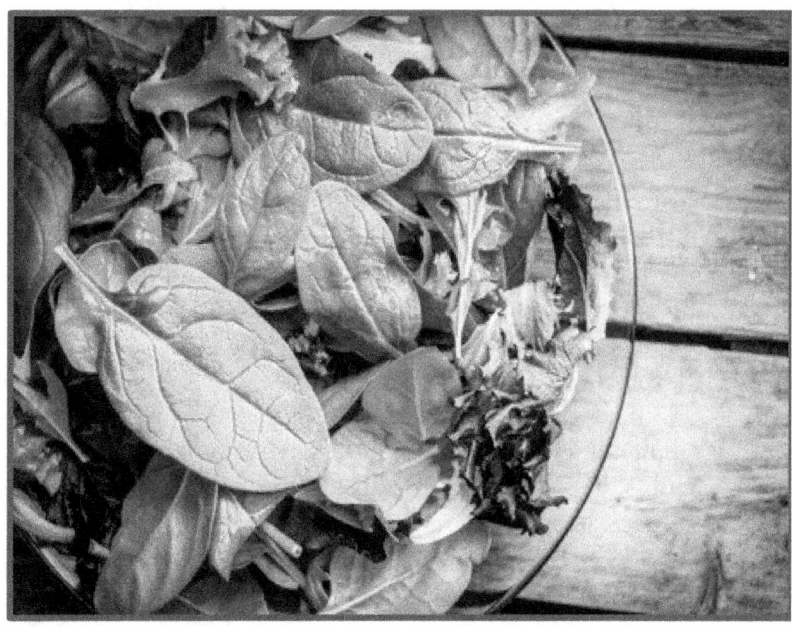

Spinach Salad with Oranges and Walnuts

To make this a complete meal, serve with a piece of lightly cooked fish, such as salmon.

INGREDIENTS:
¼ cup olive oil
¼ cup fresh orange juice
3 spring onions, white and green parts, very finely chopped
3 tablespoons white grape vinegar
1 tablespoon honey
1 teaspoon orange zest, finely grated
Salt and pepper to taste
4 medium oranges, peeled and segmented
About 180g baby spinach
2/3 cup walnuts

INSTRUCTIONS:
To make the dressing, whisk together the olive oil, orange juice, onions, vinegar, honey, and zest. Season with salt and pepper. On a serving platter, arrange your spinach leaves in a pile, then top them with orange segments. Sprinkle with the walnuts, and drizzle with the dressing.

Serves 6

Modern Cobb Salad

Always a favorite and a complete meal in itself, Cobb salad is usually very rich and full of things one shouldn't have if one is trying to eat healthily. This updated version retains all the flavor and creaminess of the classic salad, but with fewer calories.

INGREDIENTS:
Handful of salad greens
½ cup chopped broccoli
½ cup cherry tomatoes, halved
2 eggs, hardboiled and chopped
1 cup cooked, cubed turkey breast
1 large avocado, peeled, pitted, and sliced
¼ cup sliced almonds
¼ cup extra-virgin olive oil
1 clove garlic, crushed
1 tablespoon horseradish
1 tablespoons Dijon mustard
2 tablespoons red wine vinegar
Salt and pepper to taste

INSTRUCTIONS:
Use an attractive serving platter, large enough to serve 2 people. Arrange the greens first on the platter, then scatter the broccoli, tomatoes, eggs, turkey, and avocado over the top. Sprinkle with the almonds. To make the dressing, whisk together the oil, garlic, horseradish, mustard, and vinegar. Season to taste. Drizzle over the salad and serve at once.

Serves 2

Two Bean Salad

INGREDIENTS:
1 red bell pepper, seeded, and diced
1 green bell pepper, seeded, and diced
1 red onion, finely chopped
1 large tomato, chopped
I can (about 410g) red kidney beans, rinsed and drained
1 can cannellini beans, rinsed and drained
1 red chili, seeded and finely chopped
Handful of fresh parsley, finely chopped
Juice of 2 limes
¼ cup extra-virgin olive oil
Sea salt and black pepper to taste

INSTRUCTIONS:
In a bowl, mix the peppers, onion, and tomato. Add the beans, chili, parsley, lime juice, and olive oil. Season to taste. Chill and leave for a few hours before serving to allow the flavors to develop.

Serves 6-8

Chopped Salad with Avocado Dressing

This lovely salad has a gorgeous, creamy dressing. To make it a more substantial meal, mix a can of tuna chunks into the salad ingredients.

INGREDIENTS:
1 ripe avocado, peeled, seeded, and mashed
½ small onion, grated
1 clove garlic, finely grated
Juice of 1 lemon
1 teaspoon honey
Salt and pepper to taste
½ English cucumber, diced
2 medium tomatoes, diced
Small bunch of spring onions, chopped (include some green parts)
1 baby gem or cos lettuce, shredded

INSTRUCTIONS:
To make the dressing, put the avocado, onion, garlic, lemon, honey and seasoning into a blender. Puree until smooth. If it's too thick, add a small amount of water to make a pourable dressing.
Mix all the salad ingredients together in a bowl, then tip out onto a serving platter. Top with the dressing and serve at once.

Serves 1-2

Japanese Inspired Salad

Light and refreshing, with a slight bite from the ginger.

INGREDIENTS:
1 small carrot, peeled and finely grated
2 tablespoons rice vinegar
1 tablespoon soy sauce
1 tablespoon sesame oil
1 tablespoon grated fresh ginger
1 teaspoon agave to sweeten
Handful of radishes, sliced
Handful of bean sprouts
1/3 English cucumber, peeled and halved lengthways, seeds removed and sliced
I orange, peeled and segmented
Salad greens, such as mizuna

INSTRUCTIONS:
To make the dressing, put the carrot, rice vinegar, soy sauce, sesame oil, ginger, and agave into a blender or a food processor, and process until smooth. Arrange the salad greens on a serving platter, then top with the radishes, sprouts, cucumber, and orange segments. Spoon the carrot dressing over the top and serve at once.

Serves 1-2

Spring Greens and Pineapple Salad

This salad is fresh, easily adaptable, quick to make, and it will keep well in the fridge for a few days without the dressing on. It contains the green superfoods kale and spinach, which are rich in so many nutrients, for example vitamins A, C, K, and also folic acid, and iron, to name a few. Turmeric is something we could all get more of, as it has powerful anti-inflammatory effects. With the addition of the chicken, it's a meal in itself, and a perfect lunch to take to work.

INGREDIENTS:

Bunch of kale, washed and tough center stem removed

Sea salt and freshly ground black pepper, to taste

Juice of 1 lemon

2 tablespoons extra-virgin olive oil

2 handfuls baby spinach leaves

1 handful fresh parsley, chopped

1 handful fresh mint, chopped

1 small ripe pineapple, peeled and chopped

2 handfuls raw, unbleached almonds, coarsely chopped

1 handful pumpkin seeds

2 chicken breast fillets, poached, cooled, and chopped

For the dressing:

5 tablespoons extra-virgin olive oil

1 teaspoon ground turmeric

2 teaspoons freshly grated ginger

Juice of 1 lemon

1 tablespoon honey or stevia

Sea salt and black pepper to taste.

INSTRUCTIONS:

Use a large bowl. First, shred the kale with a sharp knife and place them in the bowl. Add a bit of salt and pepper, the lemon juice and oil, and leave to marinate and soften the kale for about 10 minutes. Put in the spinach, parsley, and mint. Add pineapple, almonds, and pumpkin seeds, and chicken. Add the dressing before serving, mixing it well through the ingredients. To make the dressing, whisk everything together in a small bowl until combined.

Serves 4

Crisp Clean Coleslaw

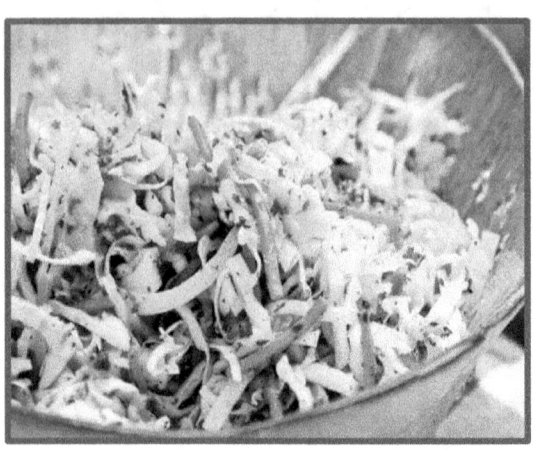

INGREDIENTS:

About 350g cabbage, finely shredded

2 large carrots, shredded

1 small red onion, finely chopped

1 green bell pepper, finely chopped

Handful fresh parsley, finely chopped

1 celery stalk, including leaves, finely chopped

Small bunch spring onions, green parts included, very finely chopped

2 tablespoons sesame seeds, lightly toasted in a dry pan

¼ cup lime juice

2 tablespoons honey

1 tablespoon apple cider vinegar

½ teaspoon ground turmeric

Sea salt and freshly ground black pepper, to taste

1 tablespoon canola oil

INSTRUCTIONS:

Using a large mixing bowl, put in the cabbage, carrots, red onion, green pepper, parsley, celery, spring onions, and sesame seeds. Mix well, using your hands. Blend the remaining ingredients together to make a dressing, tasting for seasoning. Mix into the salad and allow to stand, covered, in the fridge for about an hour before serving to allow the cabbage to soften and the flavors to blend. This salad keeps well for about 3 days in the fridge.

DINNERS

Not many of us have hours and hours after work to prepare dinner. Yet a healthy, substantial meal is still so welcome. Before you resort to unhealthy takeaways, here are some simple, fairly quick recipes that you can whip up in next to no time. It's a good idea to plan your week's menu ahead of time, so that you can buy everything ahead of time and make sure you have what you need.

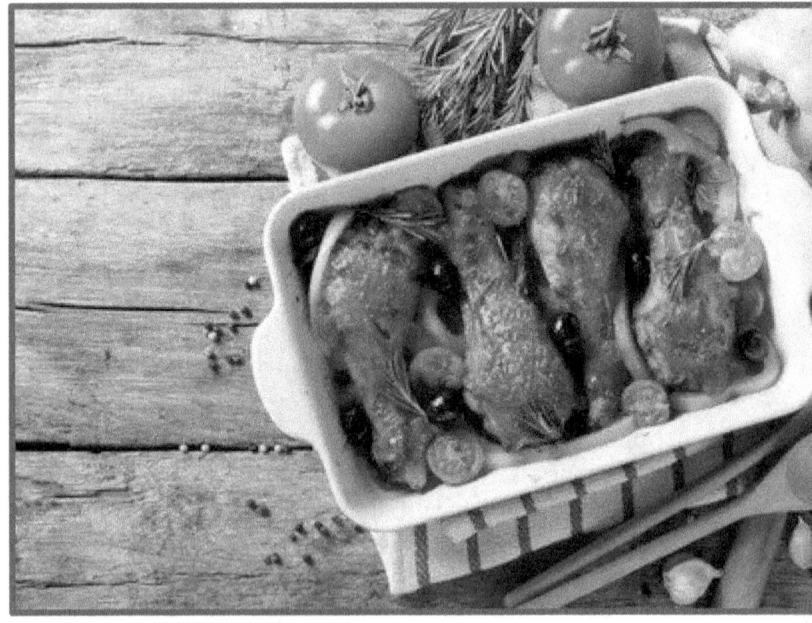

Baked Chicken

This is a wonderful all-in-one dish that can be assembled in the evening before going to bed, then refrigerating. When you come home from work the next day all you have to do is heat the oven and bake it. Miso is great for the digestion, and contains beneficial probiotics, so give it a try.

INGREDIENTS:

1½ cups chicken stock

1 tablespoon fresh thyme leaves

Juice of 2 lemons

1½ tablespoons miso paste

2 garlic cloves, crushed

1 large onion, sliced

700g sweet potatoes, sliced

5 large carrots, peeled and sliced

200g fresh green beans, topped and tailed and cut in half

6–8 organic boneless, skinless chicken breast fillets

3 tablespoons olive oil

Handful fresh parsley, chopped

¼ teaspoon cayenne pepper

INSTRUCTIONS:

Preheat oven to 220°C.

In a small bowl, mix the chicken stock, thyme, lemon juice, miso paste, and garlic. Arrange the sliced vegetables in a 3 x 22-cm baking dish. Place chicken breasts on top in a single layer. Pour stock mixture over everything, and sprinkle with the oil, parsley, and cayenne pepper. Cover with foil, shiny side facing the chicken, and bake for about an hour, turning the chicken halfway through. Serve hot with brown rice.

Serves 6.

Shrimp Pasta

INGREDIENTS:
1 tablespoon olive oil
1 tablespoon butter
1 small onion, finely chopped
1 clove garlic, finely chopped
2 medium red bell peppers, seeded and chopped
¼ cup white wine
¼ cup chicken stock
2 lemon juice
250g shrimp, peeled and deveined
200g whole-wheat pasta such as spaghetti or linguine, cooked in salted boiling water
2 tablespoons chopped parsley
A few lemon slices, for garnish
Salt and black pepper, to season.

INSTRUCTIONS:
Using a wok or large frying pan, heat the olive oil and butter. Add onion, garlic and red peppers, and sauté for a couple minutes until softened. Add white wine, chicken stock, and lemon juice. Simmer gently for a few minutes. Add shrimp, and cook for a few more minutes or until shrimp turn pink. Take off the stove, and add to the pasta, adding the parsley and seasoning of needed. Mix gently together. Serve in bowls garnished with lemon slices.

Serves 2

Thai Red Curry

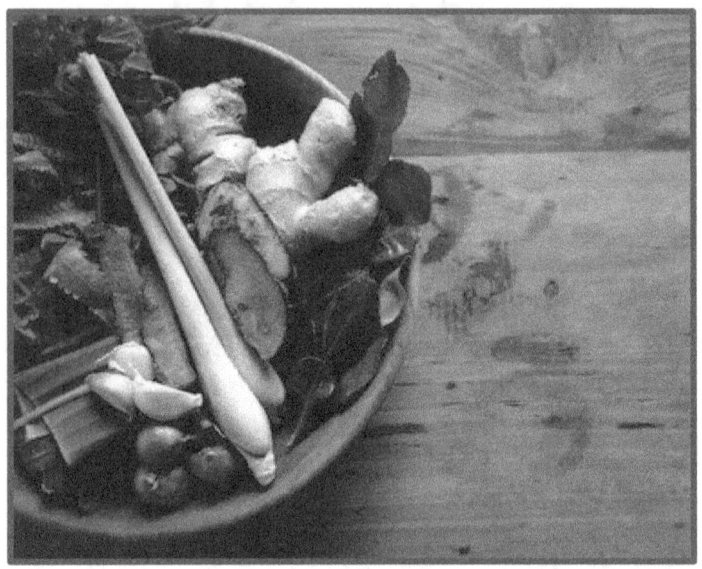

This is a delicious,exotic sounding vegetarian dish that's sure to impress any guests you may have,but is actually really easy to make.

A bonus is that it's all made in one wok, so there's less washing up afterwards! Pumpkin is highly nutritious, and is a great in

source of many vitamins and minerals,offering beta-carotene,potassium, pro-vitamin A, vitamin C,and fiber.

INGREDIENTS:

1 ½ cups coconut milk

1-2 tablespoons Thai red curry paste, depending on how hot you like your curry

1 onion, chopped

170g pumpkin, peeled and chopped

140g green beans, chopped

1 red bell pepper, seeded and chopped

3 zucchinis, chopped

1 can bamboo shoots, drained and sliced in half

2 tablespoons fresh basil leaves, shredded

2 tablespoons lemon juice

2 teaspoons agave syrup

INSTRUCTIONS:

Using a wok, put the coconut milk, curry paste, and ½ cup water into it. Bring to the boil, stirring.

Add the onion and allow to boil for a few minutes. Add the pumpkin to the wok and simmer over medium heat until nearly cooked. Add beans, red bell pepper, and zucchini, and simmer for another 5

minutes. Add water if the sauce becomes too thick. Add the shoots and basil and carry on cooking until they're heated through. Add the lemon juice and agave syrup. Check the seasoning, adding salt if necessary.

Serve on brown rice.

Serves 6.

Curried Potatoes in Tomato Sauce with Eggs

INGREDIENTS:

900g potatoes, washed and cubed

½ teaspoon salt

2 ½ cm fresh ginger

2 cloves garlic

1 onion, finely chopped

2 tablespoon olive oil

2 tablespoons mild curry powder curry powder

1 can tomato chopped tomatoes (410g)

4 eggs

INSTRUCTIONS:

Use a large pot. Put the potato cubes in with the salt and cover with water. Bring to the boil, then simmer until the potatoes are cooked. Drain. For the sauce, peel the ginger and grate it finely. Grate the garlic too. Using a big pot or large frying pan, heat the oil. Add the onion, ginger and garlic. Sauté over medium heat for a couple of minutes, being careful not to scorch it. Stir in the curry powder, and stir until fragrant.

Add the can of tomato to the pan and stir to mix. Heat until the sauce is bubbling. Taste the sauce and add salt, if needed, and a teaspoon of honey if the tomatoes are sour. Add the potatoes to the sauce and stir to coat. Add a few tablespoons of water if the mixture seems too dry.

Create four small wells in the potato mixture with a small ladle and crack an egg into each. Place a lid on the pan and let it come up to a simmer. Simmer the eggs in the sauce for about 6-8 minutes, until cooked through (less time if runny yolks are desired). Serve immediately.

Serves 2

Turkey Bolognese

Similar to the traditional Bolognese, this take on it uses lean and healthy turkey meat instead of beef.

2 tablespoons extra-virgin olive oil
1 medium onion, finely chopped
2 cloves garlic, very finely chopped
1 large green pepper, seeded and finely chopped
1 carrot, finely grated
1 stick of celery, leaves included, finely chopped
500g lean ground turkey
1 large (790g) can tomatoes, with juice, roughly chopped
1 tablespoon tomato paste
1 teaspoon dried oregano
Salt and black pepper, to taste
1 teaspoon honey or agave
¼ cup milk
300g whole-wheat spaghetti noodles, cooked in salted water

Using a large frying pan, heat the olive oil. Add the onion, garlic, and green pepper, and stir fry till softened.
Add the carrot, celery and the turkey meat, frying until brown and breaking up the lumps as you go. Add the tomatoes, tomato paste, oregano, and seasoning. Simmer, uncovered, until the sauce has thickened and

looks rich and delicious. Taste and add honey if needed to balance any sourness from the tomatoes, and add the milk for creaminess. Simmer for a further 10 minutes, and in the meantime cooking the pasta.
Serve the sauce hot over the pasta.

Serves 4-6

Roasted Chicken with Lemon, Baby Potatoes, and Broccoli

This makes a lovely roast dinner, with minimal preparation. If you don't have fresh herbs, feel free to substitute with 1 teaspoon each of dried ones.

INGREDIENTS:
1 whole organic chicken, rinsed and dried
2 tablespoons extra-virgin olive oil plus a little more for dressing the broccoli
1 handful fresh thyme, leaves picked
1 handful fresh oregano, leaves picked
2 lemons
1 teaspoon sea salt
1 teaspoon freshly ground black pepper
1 onion, chopped
About 2 dozen new (baby) potatoes
½ cup water
4 cups broccoli spears
4 sprigs parsley, chopped

INSTRUCTIONS:

Preheat the oven to 180°C. Lightly oil a small roasting pan with half the oil. In a small bowl, combine 1 tablespoon of the olive oil with the thyme, oregano, juice from one lemon, and seasoning. Save the squeezed out lemon rind. Rub the chicken with the herb mixture and place the squeezed lemon remains in the cavity of the chicken. The rind will add flavor from the inside out. Place the chopped onion on the bottom of the roasting pan, and put the chicken on top. Scatter the baby potatoes around the sides. Cover with foil (shiny side in) and roast the chicken for an hour. Remove the foil in the last 15 min so the chicken can brown. Cook for longer if the chicken is not yet done. While that's going on, steam the broccoli. Drain, then dress the broccoli with a little more olive oil, the juice of the other lemon, and the parsley.

Allow the chicken to rest in a warm place for 10 minutes before carving. Serve hot with the broccoli, new potatoes, and the onions from the roasting pan.

Serves 6

Cinnamon Baked Lamb with Butternut Squash

Warm and comforting, this dish is best served in fall or winter.

INGREDIENTS:

2 tablespoons extra-virgin olive oil

2 teaspoons ground cinnamon

1 tablespoon dried thyme

1 clove garlic, crushed

Salt and black pepper, to taste

4 lamb shanks

1 large onion, finely chopped

1 cup carrot dice

1 butternut squash, peeled, and cut into large dice

¾ cup water or red wine

INSTRUCTIONS:

Preheat the oven to 180°C and lightly oil a baking dish.

In a bowl, mix the rest of the oil with the cinnamon, thyme, garlic, and seasoning. Rub this mixture onto the lamb.

Put the onion, carrots, and butternut on the bottom of the baking dish. Put the lamb shanks on top of the vegetables. Pour in the water. Cover the dish with foil, shiny side facing the lamb, and cook the lamb for about an hour, or until tender, then remove the foil and cook, uncovered, for a further 20 minutes.

Serve with peas and mashed sweet potatoes.

Serves 4

Chicken and Mushroom Pilaf

Similar to a risotto, but with much less stirring! The rosemary blends so well with the earthy flavor of the brown rice and mushrooms.

INGREDIENTS:

3 tablespoons olive or canola oil

1 large onion, chopped

1 clove garlic, finely chopped

250g button mushrooms

Small handful fresh parsley, finely chopped

1 tablespoon fresh rosemary, chopped

1 ½ cups brown rice

3 cups chicken or stock

4 chicken breast fillets, cubed

INSTRUCTIONS:

Using a large saucepan over medium heat, heat half the olive oil. Add onion and garlic, and fry until softened. Add mushrooms and fry until most of their water has evaporated. Add the rice, and the stock, bring to a boil, and turn heat down to medium-low. Simmer for about 30 minutes or until stock has been absorbed. Stir now and again to prevent sticking. Add more stock if needed. Add the fresh herbs in the final 10 minutes of cooking.

Also in the final 10 minutes, heat the remaining oil in a separate pan, and fry the chicken cubes over high heat until just done and golden. To serve, mix the chicken through the rice and serve hot.

Serves 4

Salmon and Zucchini with Lemon and Herbs

This dinner is all made in one pan, so you won't have much washing up to do.

INGREDIENTS:

4 zucchinis, sliced in half lengthways

2 tablespoons olive oil

Sea salt and freshly ground black pepper, to taste

2 teaspoons agave

2 tablespoons lemon juice

2 cloves garlic, very finely chopped

1 tablespoon fresh dill, chopped

1 tablespoon fresh oregano, chopped

½ tablespoon fresh thyme leaves

2 tablespoons fresh parsley, chopped

Sea salt and freshly ground black pepper, to taste

4 (120-150g each) salmon fillets

INSTRUCTIONS:

Preheat oven to 200°C. Lightly oil a baking sheet.

Beat together the honey or agave, lemon juice, garlic, dill, oregano, thyme and parsley. Season with salt and pepper.

Place zucchini in a single layer onto the prepared baking sheet. Drizzle with olive oil and season with salt and pepper. Put salmon in a single layer on top and brush each salmon fillet with the herb mix.

Put into the oven and bake until the fish is done- when it flakes easily with a fork, which should take around 20 minutes. Serve at once.

Serves 4

Basic Stir-Fry

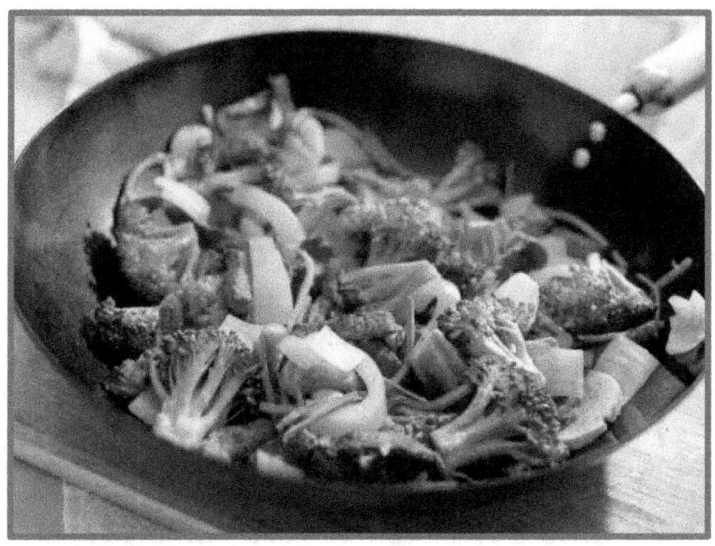

Stir fries are one of the quickest, easiest, and most nutritious meals you can make. Vary the vegetables and choice of meats each time and you'll never become tired of them.

SUGGESTED INGREDIENTS:

Vegetables such as cabbage, green beans, snap peas, bell peppers, onions, mushrooms, carrots, leeks, and zucchini.

Meats such as chicken or turkey breast, or lean pork, cut into strips (optional)

Seasonings such as soy sauce, ginger, garlic, sea salt and pepper

Oil to fry such as sesame or light olive oil.

Base to serve it on such as brown rice, gluten free noodles or rice noodles

INSTRUCTIONS:

Shred or cut all the vegetables into uniform sized strips or slices. Heat a little oil in a wok, and stir fry the vegetables until crisp-tender. Season and remove to a bowl. Wipe out the wok, add a little more oil, and stir fry the meat strips until browned. Season. Add the vegetables back to the wok and mix all together.

Meanwhile, prepare your rice or noodles. Serve with the stir-fry.

As far as quantities go, you'll need a couple of big handfuls of vegetable strips for each person, and about 100g of meat each. Remember that that vegetables reduce in volume a lot when they cook down.

Pan-Fried Salmon on Rocket Salad

INGREDIENTS:

4 salmon fillets, about 150g each

3 tablespoons fresh lemon juice

4 tablespoons extra-virgin olive oil

Salt and freshly ground black pepper, to taste

6 cups baby rocket leaves

1 ½ cups cherry tomatoes, halved

2 small red onions, thinly sliced

Salt and freshly ground black pepper, to taste

1 tablespoon balsamic vinegar

INSTRUCTIONS:

Place the salmon fillets in a shallow dish. Pour the lemon juice and 3 tablespoons of the oil over them. Season with salt and pepper and leave to one side for 15 minutes or so.

Heat a non-stick pan on medium high heat. Pan fry the fish for just a couple of minutes on each side to sear it. Lower the heat to medium, cover the pan and cook for a further 3 minutes or so, by which point the fish should be cooked through. Don't overcook it. Set aside and keep warm.

Put the rocket, tomatoes and onions into a bowl. To serve, season the salad with salt and pepper, and dress with the remaining olive oil and the vinegar.

Serves 4

Nonna's Stew

You'll love this comforting Italian vegetable stew, which brings all the flavors of Italy right into your kitchen.

INGREDIENTS:

1/2 lb. eggplant, unpeeled and cubed

2 tablespoons extra-virgin olive oil
1 large onion, thinly sliced
3 cloves garlic, crushed

1 celery stalk, finely chopped

Handful of fresh basil, stems removed, chopped
400g can Italian tomatoes, crushed

1 tablespoon tomato paste
320g potatoes, washed and cubed

225g zucchini, cut into thick rounds

1 large red bell pepper, seeded and cubed

Salt and freshly-ground black pepper

INSTRUCTIONS:

Place the eggplant cubes in a colander with a tablespoon of sea salt. Leave it over a bowl for about 20 minutes to extract any bitter juices. Rinse under running water, drain, and pat dry.
Using a large pot, heat the olive oil. Add the onion, garlic, and celery. Stir-fry over medium heat for about 5 minutes, until the vegetables have softened. Add the eggplant, and stir-fry until beginning to stick. Add the basil and the tomatoes. When it starts simmering, add the potatoes. Stir, bring to a boil, then turn down and simmer, covered, for about 15 minutes. Add the zucchini and peppers and simmer for another 15 minutes or so, until all of the vegetables are soft. Check the seasoning, adding salt and pepper if needed, and a teaspoonful of honey if the tomatoes are sour. Allow to sit in the warmer for 20 minutes or so before serving, to allow the flavors to develop.

Serves 4

SWEET TREATS

Yes, despite making the switch to an anti-inflammatory lifestyle, you can still have a few sweet treats now and again. Here, applesauce is used in baked goods instead of butter and too much sugar, and natural sweeteners like honey, agave, and maple syrup take care of that sweet tooth.

Strawberry Banana Frozen Yogurt

INGREDIENTS:

¼ cup almond or rice milk

3 ripe bananas, peeled and sliced

1 ½ cups fresh strawberries, sliced

½ cup plain low-fat Greek yogurt

INSTRUCTIONS:

Heat the milk in a saucepan over low heat, stirring until just warm. Take off the heat and mix in the honey. Put the bananas, strawberries, and yogurt in a blender and blend until smooth. Divide the mixture among four plastic cups. Place a plastic spoon into each one. Freeze until firm.

Serves 4

Oatmeal Cashew Cookies

INGREDIENTS:

1 tablespoons softened coconut butter

1/2 cup agave nectar

1/4 cup applesauce, unsweetened

1 egg

1 teaspoon vanilla extract

1 cup oats

¾ cup sorghum flour

¼ teaspoon salt

½ teaspoon baking powder

½ teaspoon baking soda

1 teaspoon ground cinnamon

¼ cup cashews, chopped

¼ cup currants

INSTRUCTIONS:

Preheat the oven to 180°C. Prepare your cookie sheet by spraying with non-stick cooking spray, or lining with baking parchment.

Stir together the coconut butter, agave nectar, applesauce, egg, and vanilla extract.

In a separate bowl, mix the oats, flour, salt, baking powder, baking soda, and cinnamon.

Gently fold the dry ingredients into the applesauce mixture and stir until just blended. Mix in the cashews and currants. Drop heaped teaspoonfuls of dough onto the baking sheet, and flatten slightly. Bake the cookies for 10 to 12 minutes or until the edges are slightly browned. Remove from oven, allow to cool for a few minutes, then place on a wire rack to finish cooling. Store in an airtight tin.

Makes about 12

Honey-Ginger Syrupy Baked Pears

The flavors of pears and ginger go so well together, while the honey adds that extra touch of sweetness you've been craving.

INGREDIENTS:

4 ripe but firm pears, peeled, cored, and halved

4 tablespoons honey

1 teaspoon cinnamon

1-inch piece fresh ginger, peeled and grated

½ cup water

¼ cup chopped nuts, such as walnuts or cashews (optional)

INSTRUCTIONS:

Preheat the oven to 180°C. Line the base of a glass ovenproof dish with baking parchment. Place the pear halves, flat side down, into the dish. Drizzle with half the honey. Bake them for about 15 minutes or until they're soft, but not mushy.

Meanwhile, make the ginger syrup. Put the ginger, water, and remaining honey into a small pot. Bring to the boil, then simmer on medium heat for about 10 minutes until it goes syrupy. Strain. Serve warm or chilled, as you prefer. To serve, place a pear on each plate and spoon some syrup over the top. Sprinkle with cinnamon and nuts, if using.

Serves 4

Crustless Apple and Cranberry Pie

Apple pie is such a classic, and this new version is full of goodness. The apples are beautifully complimented by the cinnamon and walnuts.

INGREDIENTS:

1 egg, well beaten

¼ cup agave syrup or honey

½ cup whole-wheat flour 1 tsp. baking powder

¼ teaspoon salt

½ teaspoon ground cinnamon

½ teaspoon vanilla extract

3 cooking apples, peeled, cored, and diced

½ cup dried cranberries

½ cup walnuts, chopped

INSTRUCTIONS:

Preheat the oven to 180°C. Spray a 25cm pie dish with cooking spray.

In a large bowl, put the beaten egg, agave syrup, flour, baking powder, salt, cinnamon, and vanilla extract, and stir together well with a wooden spoon.

Add apples, cranberries, and walnuts, and mix well. Don't worry if the mixture looks lumpy. Pour into the prepared dish, and bake for 30 minutes.

Serve warm or cool.

Servings-4

Raisin and Spice Cookies

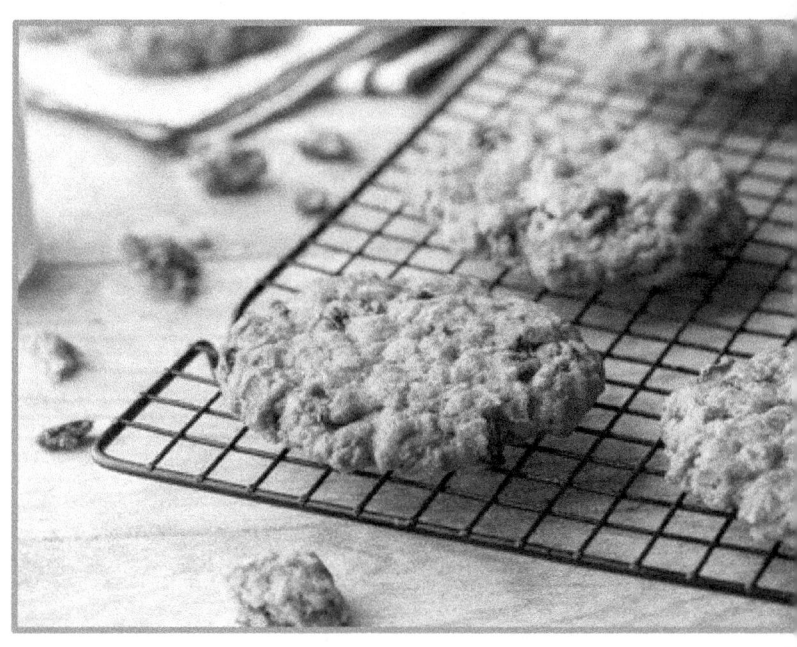

INGREDIENTS:

1½ cup spelt flour

1 cup oat flour

2 teaspoons baking powder

1 teaspoon baking soda

2 teaspoons ground cinnamon

2 teaspoons ground ginger

2/3 cup raisins

90ml coconut oil, melted

3 tablespoons rice or almond milk

1½ cups grated carrots

½ cup honey

1 egg

Pinch of salt

INSTRUCTIONS:

Preheat the oven to 180° C. Prepare a baking sheet by lining it with baking parchment, or greasing it with coconut oil.

Mix all the dry ingredients together. In a large bowl, mix all the liquid ingredients together. Add the carrots. Add the dry ingredients, mixing well. Drop with a spoonfuls onto the baking sheet and bake for about 8-10 minutes.

Makes about 35 cookies.

Oat Cookies

INGREDIENTS:

1 egg, beaten

¼ cup rice or almond milk

1 cup coconut oil, melted

½ cup honey

1 teaspoon vanilla extract

1½ cups oat flour

1 teaspoon baking soda

1 teaspoon cinnamon

1 teaspoon sea salt

3 cups rolled oats

½ cup walnuts, chopped

¼ cup sunflower seeds

½ cup apple, peeled and grated

INSTRUCTIONS:

Preheat oven to 180° C. Prepare a baking sheet by lining it with baking parchment.

In a big bowl, mix together wet ingredients. In another bowl, mix together the oat flour, baking soda, cinnamon, and salt. Mix the two mixtures together till you have a smooth batter. Add oats, nuts, seeds,

and apple, stirring until combined. Drop spoonfuls onto the prepared cookie sheet, and bake for about 10 minutes.

Makes about 25 cookies.

Minty Berry Sorbet

Substitute frozen grated pineapple and mango for the berries in this dessert if you like, to make a tropical flavored sorbet, and use coconut milk instead of rice milk.

INGREDIENTS:

2 cups frozen berries, such as blueberries or strawberries

¼ cup rice milk

2 tablespoons honey or maple syrup

1 tablespoon lemon juice

Small handful of mint leaves, picked off the stem and finely chopped

INSTRUCTIONS:

Put the frozen fruit in a blender and add the rice milk. Add honey or maple syrup, lemon juice, and blend until the mixture reaches a smooth consistency. Garnish with a sprig of mint and serve at once in small dessert bowls.

Serves 4.

Conclusion

Well, it was great to end the book off on a sweet note. I hope you'll come back to these recipes again and again as you embrace a healthier way of eating.

Starting a new way of eating can seem overwhelming at first, as we are conditioned from childhood and by the culture surrounding us in a certain way. Just remember to start off slowly, making small changes in your diet one at a time, and your new anti-inflammatory way of eating will soon become a way of life that you can pass on to future generations.

You could start off by eliminating any foods that you know have a bad effect on your digestion, such as gluten or dairy, perhaps. Moving on from there, you can make small substitutions, replacing milk chocolate with dark, white bread with oat bread, and white rice with brown. You can then go on to increase your intake of fresh vegetables, perhaps cooking just one extra vegetable at dinner, or starting off dinner with a soup or a salad. Takeaway meals at lunch can then be substituted with filling salads or soup in a flask, and you'll probably find that everyone at your place of work will want some too!

After that, you can focus on breakfast, stocking up on simple fruits and yoghurt to make quick and filling smoothies, and as a contrast, having a breakfast of eggs a few times a week too.

Have a look at your drinks throughout the day, too, making sure that your main source of liquid is water. Flavor it with mint, ginger, or slices of citrus fruit if you find plain water unpalatable. Eliminate sodas and fruit punches, instead having herbal teas which come in so many flavors you're sure to find one you like. Chai teas are lovely for winter, with their warm spicy flavors they're sure to warm you up.

I wish you all the best on this journey, remember that it's a marathon not a sprint, so pace yourself and be kind to yourself, allowing for the occasional slip. After a short time, you'll start to feel the benefits, reaping the reward of increased energy, a reduction in symptoms of chronic illness you may have, fewer colds and infections, and clear glowing skin and eyes.

Enjoy the journey!

A Leptin Mediterranean Diet

Exploration Over 50 Enticing Recipes To Energise Your Day

and Excite Your Palate

By: Emily Simmons

Introduction

So, what exactly is "Leptin-Mediterranean" anyway?

Leptin is a little molecule, a hormone actually, that is responsible for controlling fat storage in our bodies. It controls which nutrients get stored as fat, and which are going to be directly used for energy. In obese people, leptin is usually in short supply, so their bodies need a nudge to produce the correct levels. Studies have shown that this "nudge" can be provided by 5 basic things:

1. Not eating after an early dinner. (Eating late causes almost every calorie consumed to be stored as fat.)
2. Eating 3 meals a day without snacking in between. The idea is to maintain 3-6 hours between meals without having other food as well. We often perceive thirst in between meals as hunger, so rather than snack, drink plenty of water.
3. Don't eat big meals. It's a misconception that people in Mediterranean regions eat huge dishes

full of pasta and meat, with big wedges of bread on the side, along with bottle after bottle of red wine. In truth, they have several small dishes, consisting mainly of fruit and vegetables with some legumes, and small amounts of meat as flavoring, with a glass of wine. But more about that just now. If our bodies are fed large amounts of food in one go, we can be sure that some of it will be stored as fat. Large meals interfere with the production of leptins by our bodies.

4. Eat a protein-rich breakfast, focusing on breakfast as the main meal of the day, rather than dinner. There's an old saying that has some wisdom, "Eat breakfast like a king, lunch like a peasant, and supper like a pauper." So, you'll find our breakfast recipes here are full of good proteins like lean ham, eggs, feta cheese, chicken breast, and lean beef. Try them, and you'll eliminate those mid-morning hunger pangs.

5. Reduce (don't eliminate) the amount of carbohydrates eaten. Our bodies are designed to

crave them for times of survival, in order to increase fat reserves, which is exactly what we don't need in these times of relative abundance. Rather fill up on fruits, vegetables, cottage cheese, yoghurts, or make some delicious healthy soups from our soup chapter.

As far as Mediterranean food goes, it is essentially balanced between the sea and the land.

I say, "From the land," because of the gorgeous olive oils, honey, nuts, vegetables, fruits, meats, and legumes that are produced; "From the sea," because the cuisine incorporates good amounts of fish and shellfish. Dishes from the Mediterranean region normally retain an essential freshness and simplicity. Food here is always more than just nourishment for the body. It is also nourishment for the soul, for family bonds, and for friendship. Even in these modern days of busyness and rush, time is still taken in the preparation of the food and the enjoyment of it. The principle of "slow food", which has become so trendy in the West, has been practiced for centuries in the Mediterranean region.

Staples in the region's kitchens are wheat (made into flour for pastas, breads, and pastries); vegetables (notably tomatoes, artichokes, courgettes, peppers, garlic, among many others); legumes (dried beans, lentils, chickpeas); and, of course, herbs and spices for flavoring all of this ((pepper, thyme, rosemary, bay, cumin, nutmeg, cinnamon etc.) Oils, too, are a staple, particularly olive. Meats are lean and are secondary to the meal- more of a flavoring than a base for the whole dish. Sweets are usually fruits, such as figs, grapes, and oranges, with the odd pastry as well. There is an emphasis on fresh, homegrown, or homemade produce, rather than processed food.

The benefits of eating this way have been known about and studied since after the Second World War, when studies were done comparing the cardio-vascular health and longevity of men in the West and those in the Mediterranean lands.

So, what we've done in this book is combine the modern principles that are known of leptin's role in weight control, with the ancient way of eating that has been practiced for centuries in the Mediterranean region that is known to promote health, and we've come up with some simple, healthy, and delicious recipes that we hope will become part of your everyday diet. So, if you want protection against type 2 diabetes, heart disease and stroke; a reduced risk of developing Alzheimer's; a decreased risk of getting Parkinson's disease; increased longevity, as well as a day filled with delicious easy-to-cook meals, then make this recipe book a part of your lifestyle!

LEPTIN-MEDITERRANEAN HEALTHY BREAKFAST RECIPES

So, let's begin at sunrise. A great breakfast is where a day full of energy begins, and where you start to beat those mid-morning hunger pangs. You should notice improved concentration for your work morning, too. We've given you a selection of quick-to-make recipes for busy weekday mornings, as well as some for the weekend when you have a little more time.

Mediterranean Ham and Egg Cups

This one's full of good things, like spinach and feta, as well as a good dose of protein from the eggs. Basil and pesto add flavour and freshness.

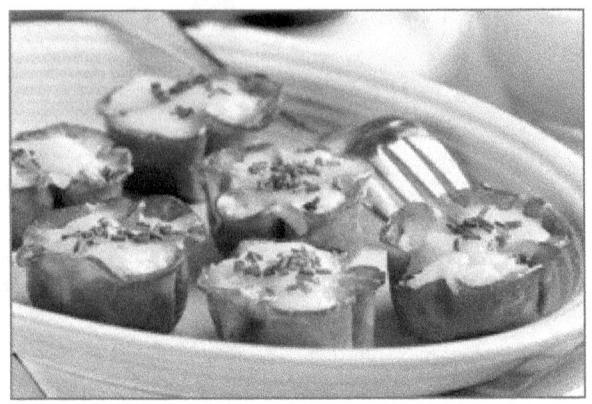

SERVES: 6

INGREDIENTS:

- 6 slices of thin cut deli ham

- 1 large red bell pepper, roasted, peeled and seeded, quartered

- 1/3 cup fresh spinach, finely chopped

- 1/4 cup low-fat feta cheese, crumbled

- 8 egg whites

- 1 large whole egg

- Salt and freshly ground black pepper, to taste

- 2 tablespoons of pesto sauce

- Oil, for greasing muffin tin

- Fresh basil leaves, for garnish

- 1 red bell pepper, roasted, peeled and seeded, quartered

DIRECTIONS:

1. Preheat oven with high heat and line a baking tray with parchment paper. Place the bell pepper on the baking tray.

2. Roast bell pepper for about 15 to 20 minutes or until the pepper starts to turn black, skin side down on the baking tray. Check the pepper regularly and remove from the oven when it starts to turn black. Set aside to cool.

3. Bring the oven temperature to 400 °F and lightly grease a muffin tin with oil.

4. Line each muffin tin with a slice of ham, making sure you don't leave spaces for the egg mix to run out.

5. Peel the skin and deseed the roasted pepper.

6. Place each slice of roasted pepper on the muffin tin together with the ham. Add 1 tablespoon of spinach on top of each pepper.

7. Top off each portion with feta cheese crumbles.

8. In a mixing bowl, combine together the egg whites, whole egg, and then season with salt and pepper. Pour into the ham cups.

9. Bake them in the oven for about 15 minutes, or until the eggs are puffy and firm. Remove muffin tin from the oven and top off with pesto sauce, extra roasted red peppers and chopped basil. Serve.

Mediterranean Chicken Quiche

Bake this lovely quiche the night before, if you're pushed for time in the morning, and tuck a slice or two into the kids' lunchboxes for school, too.

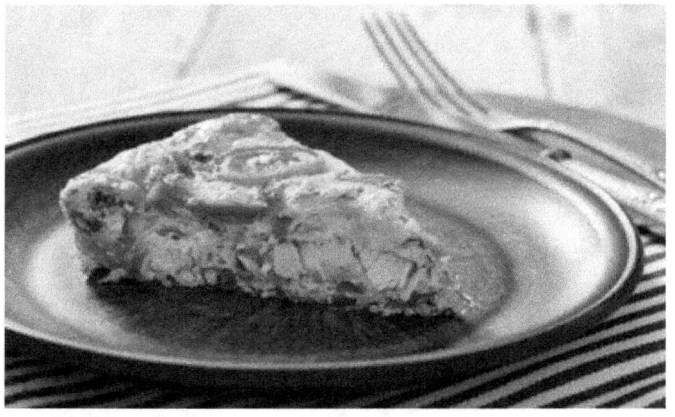

SERVES: 6

INGREDIENTS:

- ½ pound cooked chicken breast, deboned and skin removed, shredded

- 1/2 cup cherry tomatoes, halved

- 1/3 cup Feta cheese, crumbled

- 1 scallion, thinly sliced

- 2 tablespoons of fresh dill, coarsely chopped

- 2 tablespoons fresh mint leaves, coarsely chopped

- 3 large eggs

- 1 cup whole milk

- 1/4 teaspoon ground nutmeg

- Salt and freshly ground black pepper, to taste

FOR THE CRUST:

2 Med - large eggs, whisked

1/3 cup coconut oil, melted

Additional coconut oil, for greasing pie plate

3/4 cup coconut flour, sifted, preferably gluten-free

DIRECTIONS:

1. Preheat an oven to 350°F and lightly grease a 9-inch pie plate. Set aside.

2. In a medium bowl, whisk 2 eggs and oil until well incorporated. Stir in flour and blend together.

3. Add flour mix to the pie plate, press mixture with your hands until base and sides of the plate are evenly covered with crust mixture.

4. Bake it in the oven for about 10 minutes, or until light brown. Remove from the oven and set aside.

5. Increase the oven temperature to 375°F.

6. In a mixing bowl, combine together the shredded chicken, cherry tomatoes, cheese, scallions, dill and mint. Place it on top of the pie shell.

7. In separate mixing bowl, whisk together 3 eggs, milk, nutmeg, salt and pepper. Whisk it thoroughly until well incorporated, pour sauce on top of the chicken-vegetable mixture and crust.

8. Bake it in the middle rack of the oven for about 30 minutes. It is ready when a cocktail stick inserted into the thick part of quiche comes out clean, about 30 minutes. Remove from the oven and let it rest to cool before serving.

Mediterranean Beef Frittata

A frittata is an Italian version of the omelette, where instead of filling the eggs with the meats and cheese, the eggs are mixed through so that the deliciousness from the filling is all over them. You're getting in some extra veg, too, which is always a good thing!

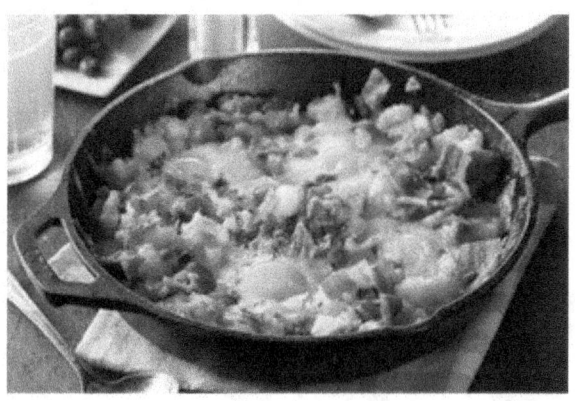

SERVES: 4

INGREDIENTS:

- 1 pound ground beef, grass-fed preferably
- 1 red bell pepper, diced
- 6 asparagus spears, chopped
- 1/2 onion, diced
- 1/2 cup canned mushrooms, quartered
- 1/2 cup arugula, chopped

- 1 tablespoon garlic, minced
- Salt and freshly ground black pepper, to taste
- 7 large eggs
- 1/4 cup milk
- 1 tablespoon of extra virgin olive oil
- 1 package of non-fat Greek yogurt (about 6 ounces)
- 1 cup Feta cheese, crumbled
- 2 tomatoes, sliced into rounds
- 1 tablespoon of dried oregano

DIRECTIONS:

1. Preheat an oven to 425°F.
2. In a pan over medium-high heat, add the oil and brown ground beef when the oil is hot, draining off any excess fat. Once beef is fully cooked and most liquid has evaporated, add the red pepper, asparagus, onions, mushrooms, arugula, garlic, season with salt and pepper. Stir to combine the ingredients evenly, cover lid and bring to a boil. Reduce to low heat and let simmer for about 10 minutes, stirring occasionally.

3. In a mixing bowl, combine together the eggs, milk, Greek yogurt and feta cheese. Whisk the ingredients thoroughly until well incorporated.

4. Lightly grease a 9-inch baking tray with oil and add in the beef and vegetable mixture. Top with egg-yogurt mixture. Give a quick stir to evenly distribute the ingredients. Garnish with sliced tomatoes and sprinkle with oregano on top.

5. Bake it in the oven for about 25 to 30 minutes, or until thoroughly cooked. It is done when a toothpick inserted in the thickest part comes out clean. Remove from oven and let it rest for about 5 to 10 minutes. Let it cool before slicing, serve with extra cheese and Greek yogurt on top.

Mediterranean Egg Muffins

Whether you call quinoa "The Gold of the Incas" or "The Supergrain of the Future", we could all do with more of it in our diets. It is a complete protein, and contains twice the fibre of other grains, as well as good amounts of iron. In fact, this recipe is chock-full of iron because parsley and egg yolks are good sources, too.

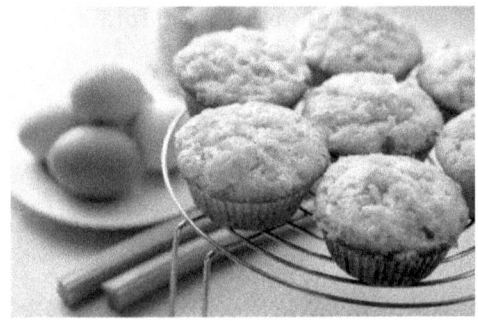

SERVES: 4

INGREDIENTS:

- 3 eggs
- 3 egg whites
- ½ cup Feta cheese, crumbled
- 1 ½ cup mixed vegetables, blanched

- 1 cup quinoa, cooked according to package directions
- 1 tablespoon onion powder
- ½ teaspoon salt, to taste
- ½ teaspoon of freshly ground black pepper, to taste
- ½ cup fresh parsley leaves, chopped
- Oil, for greasing

DIRECTIONS:

1. Preheat oven to 340°F. Lightly grease a muffin tin with oil and set aside.
2. In a mixing bowl, whisk together the eggs and egg whites for about 2 minutes or until soft peaks form.
3. Add the cheese, vegetables, quinoa, onion powder, season with salt and pepper, mix well to combine.
4. Fill each muffin tin with the mixture and bake for about 25 minutes, or until golden brown.
5. Sprinkle with chopped fresh parsley on top, let it rest to cool then serve.

Mediterranean Vegetable Cakes

Full of Mediterranean flavours such as olives, tomatoes, and artichokes, these yummy fritters are bound to become a favourite.

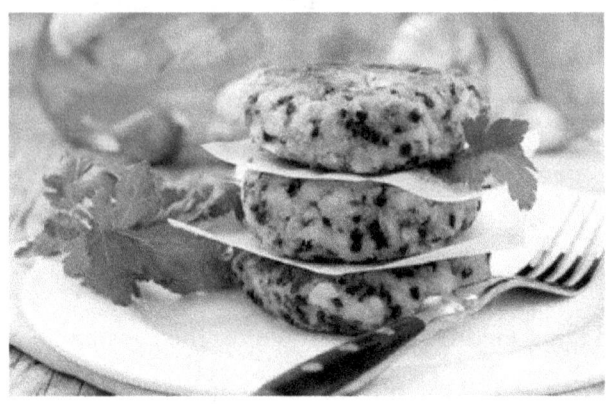

SERVES: 4

INGREDIENTS:

- 2 tablespoons of extra-virgin olive oil
- 1 medium sweet onion, diced
- 2 garlic cloves, minced
- 3 cups baby spinach,
- 1 large parsnip, peeled and grated
- 1 teaspoon of dried oregano leaves

- ¼ cup tomatoes, sun-dried, chopped
- ¼ cup Kalamata olives, chopped
- ¼ cup artichoke hearts, chopped
- 2 large eggs, lightly beaten
- ¼ cup almond flour, sifted
- ½ teaspoon of salt, to taste
- ¼ teaspoon freshly ground black pepper, to taste

DIRECTIONS:

1. Add 1 tablespoon of oil to a frying pan and place on a medium heat, once the oil is hot, add the onions and sauté until translucent and soft, stirring frequently for about 3 to 5 minutes. Add in the garlic and sauté for another minute.

2. Add the spinach, stir occasionally cooking until soft. Take off the heat and transfer it in a large bowl.

3. Stir in the grated parsnips, dried oregano, beaten eggs, sun-dried tomatoes, olives, artichokes, almond flour, and then season with black pepper and salt. Blend the ingredients well to combine. Set aside.

4. Divide the mixture into 4 equal portions.

5. In the same skillet over medium heat, add in the remaining oil. When the oil is hot, fry cakes in the skillet for 5-7 minutes on either side, or until golden and crispy. Flip it over and cook the other side for about 4 to 5 minutes.

6. Transfer it on a serving dish and serve hot. Pair with olive tapenade or mojo verde.

Mediterranean Breakfast Sandwiches

Sandwiches for breakfast? Of course, especially when they're made with toast and eggs. You won't need anything else before lunchtime after one of these.

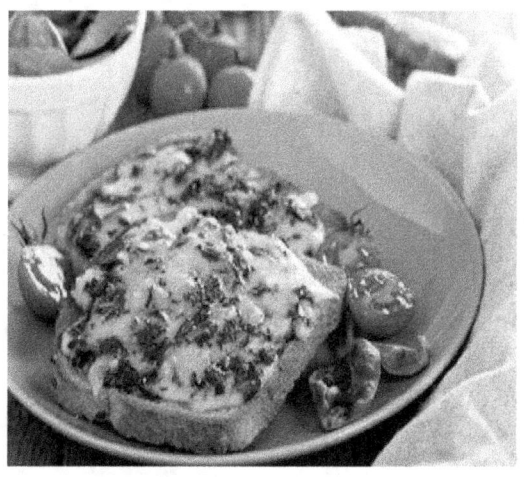

SERVES: 4

INGREDIENTS:

- 4 thin slices of multigrain sandwich

- 4 teaspoons of extra virgin olive oil

- 1 tablespoon fresh rosemary

- 4 eggs

- 2 cups fresh baby spinach leaves, blanched

- 1 medium tomato, cut into 8 thin round slices

- ¼ cup of reduced-fat Feta cheese, crumbled

- 1/8 teaspoon salt, to taste

- 1/8 teaspoon of freshly ground black pepper, to taste

DIRECTIONS:

1. Preheat oven to 375 °F.

2. Divide each sandwich into two. Set aside the half and lightly brush the other half of sandwich with olive oil. Place it on a baking sheet and toast it in the oven for about 5 minutes, or until the edges are crisp and light brown. Remove from the oven and set it aside.

3. While toasting the bread slices, heat the remaining oil in a large skillet over medium-high heat.

Add the rosemary and break the eggs, cook one at a time in the skillet. Cook for about a minute or until the egg white is cooked, but the egg yolk is still runny. Remove from skillet and continue to cook the remaining eggs. Break the egg yolks, flip it over to cook the other side for another minute, or until cooked through. Remove the skillet from heat and set aside.

4. Portion the toasted sandwich on four individual serving plates. Divide the blanched baby spinach into 4 equal portions and add it on top of the sandwich. Top off each slice of sandwich with tomato slices, 1 egg, and a tablespoon of crumbled Feta cheese. Season with the salt and pepper to taste. Top with the remaining sandwich thin halves.

Potato Hash with Chickpea

You'll just have one pan to wash after making this spicy hash, flavoured with curry and ginger, and guaranteed to wake your taste buds up! Protein from the eggs and chickpeas sets you up for the day.

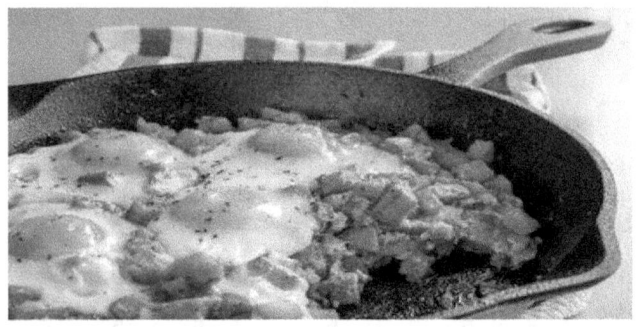

SERVES: 4 to 6

INGREDIENTS:

- 4 cups hash brown potatoes, frozen and shredded

- 2 cups baby spinach, finely chopped

- ½ cup onion, diced

- 1 tablespoon of fresh ginger root, minced
- 1 tablespoon curry powder
- salt, to taste
- ¼ cup extra-virgin olive oil
- 2 cups of canned chickpeas, rinsed and drained
- 1 large zucchini, finely chopped
- 4 large eggs

Instructions:

1. In a large bowl, combine together the shredded hash browns, chopped spinach, onion, curry powder, minced ginger, and season with salt.
2. In a non-stick skillet, heat in the oil on a medium to high heat. Drop in the potato mixture and compress into an even layer. Fry, without mixing, until the bottom is crisp and golden, this will take around 4 minutes. Once crisp turn it over and for a further 2 or 3 minutes.

3.	Turn down the heat to medium-low and fold in the zucchini with the chickpeas, separating any large pieces of potato and combine the ingredients well. Press down with a wooden spoon to form a smooth layer. Make or provide 4 spaces like a well in the base for the eggs. Break the eggs, individually into a cup, carefully place it in the space provided. Continue the process with the other eggs. Place a lid over the top and cook the eggs to your preferred taste, this will take around 4 to 5 minutes.

Banana Nut Oatmeal

Quick and easy for those days when you have to rush, but don't want to compromise on good nutrition. Flaxseeds come with a host of benefits, some of them being an ability to improve blood pressure, lower fasting-glucose levels, and decrease central obesity (that "bad fat" around the waistline.) Crush them first for maximum benefit.

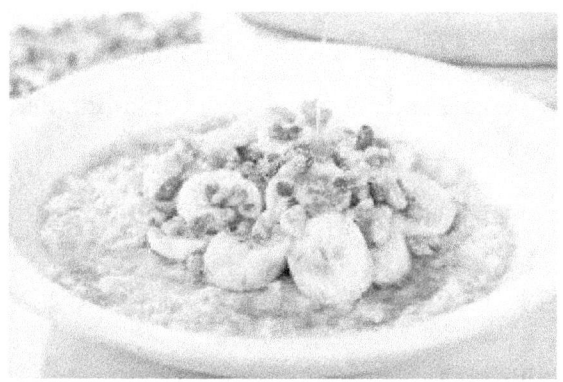

SERVES: 4

INGREDIENTS:

- ¼ cup of quick cooking oats

- ½ cup of skim milk

- 1 teaspoon flax seeds

- 2 tablespoons of walnuts, chopped

- 3 tablespoons of local honey

- 1 ripe banana, peeled and sliced into thin rounds

DIRECTIONS:

1. In a microwaveable container, combine the oats, flax seeds, banana and chopped walnuts. Stir in milk and honey.
2. Mash the banana with a fork and add it with the mixture. Mix it thoroughly to combine the ingredients.
3. Cook in microwave on high for 2 minutes. Serve warm with whipped cream or Greek yogurt.

Melamen

Melamen is a little-known Mediterranean-style stir fry. I think of this version as an upside-down omelette!

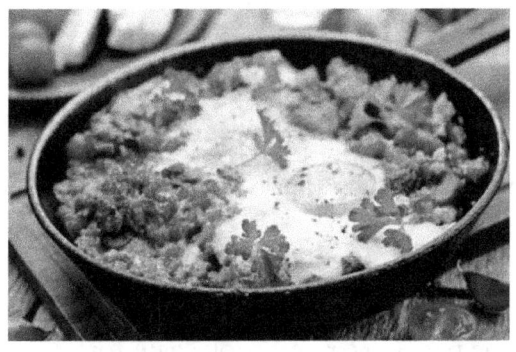

SERVES: 4

INREDIENTS:

- 1 tablespoon of extra-virgin olive oil

- 2 green bell peppers, diced

- 2 small onions, diced

- 4 medium tomatoes, diced

- 2 egg

- ½ teaspoon of salt and black pepper, to taste

- Fresh parsley leaves, for garnish

DIRECTIONS:

1. In a pan over high heat, add the olive oil and cook the green peppers for 2 minutes, covered. Reduce to medium heat and cook for another 3 minutes, or until soft.
2. While cooking the bell pepper, dice the onions and stir them into the pan. Cover and cook again for another 1 to 2 minutes.
3. Dice the tomatoes and stir it in the pan when the onion is soft and translucent. Season with salt and pepper. Cover lid, reduce to low heat.
4. Simmer for 15 minutes with cover or until the tomatoes are soft and the melamen is still juicy. Remove pan from heat, and let the melamen rest in the pan to continue the cooking process with the heat from the pan.
5. Beat the eggs and gently pour them over the top of the melamen. Do not touch or stir the melamen, but allow the egg to be cooked on top. Serve warm.

Mediterranean Chicken Stir-Fry

This would work for dinner, too. Or lunch for that matter...Barley is good for keeping your blood sugar levels stable through the day. Studies done in Japan showed that regular barley intake significantly reduced serum cholesterol and visceral fat, both accepted markers of cardiovascular risk.

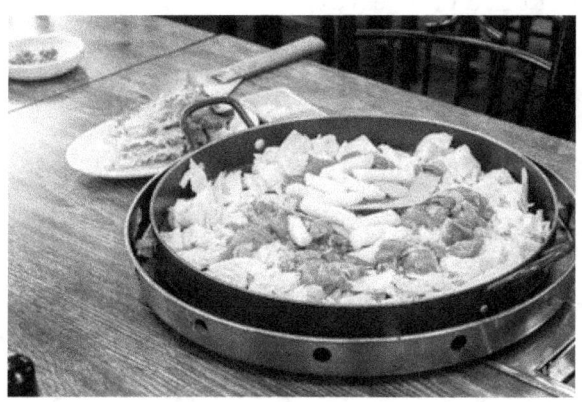

SERVES: 4

INGREDIENTS:

- 2 cups of water
- 1 cup quick-cooking barley

- 1 pound chicken breasts, deboned and skin removed, cubed
- 3 teaspoons of olive oil extra-virgin, divided
- 1 medium onion, diced
- 2 medium zucchini, cubed
- 2 garlic cloves, minced
- 1 teaspoon of dried oregano
- ½ teaspoon of dried basil leaves
- ¼ teaspoon salt, to taste
- ¼ teaspoon freshly ground black pepper, to taste
- A pinch of red pepper flakes, crushed
- 2 plum tomatoes, diced
- ½ cup pitted Greek olives, quartered
- 1 tablespoon freshly chopped parsley

DIRECTIONS:

1. In a small saucepan or pot high heat, insert the water and bring it to a boil. Stir in the barley and cover with lid. Reduce to low heat and simmer for about 10 to 12 minutes, or until barley is tender. Remove pan or pot from heat, set aside and let it stand for 5 minutes.

2. While simmering the liquid, add in 2 teaspoons of oil in a large skillet or wok. Once the oil is hot, stir-fry chicken pieces until no longer pink. Remove from wok and keep warm.

3. Stir-fry onion in remaining oil for 3 minutes. Add the zucchini, garlic, basil, oregano, seasoning and pepper flakes; stir-fry 2-4 minutes longer or until vegetables are crisp-tender. Add the chicken, olives, tomatoes, and parsley. Dish up with barley.

LEPTIN MEDITERRANEAN HEALTHY LUNCH RECIPES

While breakfast may be the most important meal of the day, lunch provides that top-up of nutrients and energy necessary to take you through the afternoon. A lunch too high in carbohydrates will cause your energy levels to plummet during the afternoon and make you sleepy, but these tasty meals will see you through the remainder of the day.

Mediterranean Salmon Salad

Try this lovely dressing with other leafy salads, too. Orzo is a quick-cooking, rice-shaped pasta, that adds a smooth texture to the salad and absorbs some of the salmon juices and delicious dressing at the same time.

SERVES: 5

INGREDIENTS:

For the Dressing

- 1/3 cup of extra-virgin olive oil
- 1/3 cup of red wine vinegar
- 1 teaspoon of dried oregano
- 1 teaspoon of onion powder
- 1/2 teaspoon of salt, to taste
- 1/2 teaspoon of freshly ground black pepper, to taste
- 1 teaspoon of Dijon mustard
- 1 teaspoon of dried basil
- 1 teaspoon of garlic powder

For the Salad

- 1 salmon filet (about ¾ pounds),
- A pinch of salt and a pinch of black pepper, to taste
- 1/4 teaspoon of dried oregano
- 1 cup dry orzo, cooked ahead according to package directions
- 1/4 cup cherry tomatoes/ olives, halved

- 1 red bell pepper, seeded and diced
- 1/2 large red onion, diced
- 1/2 cup of Feta cheese, crumbled/ Mozzarella, shredded
- 1 1/2 cups of canned artichoke hearts, drained and quartered
- 5 cups mixed leafy greens

DIRECTIONS:

1. In a mixing bowl, whisk together all ingredients except for the oil until all ingredients are well incorporated. Gradually add in small amounts of olive oil and continue to whisk until you have a thick and smooth consistency.
2. Preheat oven to 425 °F. Line a baking sheet with foil and lightly grease with oil.
3. Place salmon on a greased baking sheet lined with foil, season with salt, black pepper and oregano.
4. Bake it in the oven for about 10 to 15 minutes, or until the center is cooked through.
5. While baking the salmon, cook orzo according to package directions. Drain orzo and transfer into a

casserole dish. Add in 1/4 cup of salad dressing in the casserole with the pasta, gently toss to combine. Stir in the tomatoes, feta, artichoke hearts, red bell peppers, red onions, mixed leafy greens, and the remaining salad dressing. Toss to gently combine all ingredients.

6. Once salmon is cooked, remove from the oven and flake salmon using two forks. Portion salad in individual serving bowls/large bowl and top off with flaked salmon.

Spinach Salad with Chicken, Avocado, and Goat Cheese

A quick and substantial salad, which is also great for in a lunchbox at work or school. Just pack the dressing separately and pour over before serving.

SERVES: 4

INGREDIENTS:

FOR THE SALAD:

- 8 cups of spinach, coarsely chopped

- 1 cup of cherry tomatoes, halved
- 1/2 cup canned corn
- 1 1/2 to 2 cups of grilled/boiled chicken
- 1 large avocado, pitted and sliced
- 1/2 cup soft goat's cheese or feta cheese, crumbled
- 1/4 cup pine nuts, toasted

DRESSING:

- 2 to 3 tablespoons of white wine vinegar
- 2 tablespoons of extra-virgin olive oil
- 1 tablespoon of Dijon mustard
- salt and freshly ground black pepper, to taste

DIRECTIONS:

1. In a large salad bowl, add all salad ingredients and gently toss to combine. Stir in cooked chicken, gently toss and set aside.

2. In a separate small bowl, whisk together the entire ingredients for the dressing. Pour dressing over the salad

and gently toss. Serve with extra toasted nuts and crumbled cheese on top.

Italian Chopped Salad Recipe

Don't let the long list of ingredients put you off. Everything is quickly chopped and tossed together. Perfect when you're having friends over. Serve with a loaf of good bread for a complete meal.

SERVES: 10

INGREDIENTS:

- 3 cups of romaine lettuce, torn
- 1 cup of canned chickpeas, rinsed and drained
- 1 jar of artichoke hearts or about 6 ounces, drained and chopped
- 1 green bell pepper, diced
- 2 medium ripe tomatoes, diced
- 1/4 cup of ripe olives, drained and halved
- 1/2 cup of deli ham, diced
- 1/2 cup of hard salami, diced
- 1/2 cup pepperoni, diced
- 1/4 cup of Provolone cheese, shredded or cubed
- 2 stems of green onions, coarsely chopped

- 1/4 cup of extra-virgin olive oil
- 2 to 3 tablespoons of red wine vinegar
- 1/4 teaspoon of salt and 1/8 teaspoon of freshly ground black pepper, to taste
- 1/4 cup of shredded Parmesan cheese

DIRECTIONS:

1. In a large mixing bowl, add in romaine lettuce, chickpeas, artichoke hearts, bell pepper, tomatoes, olives, ham, salami, pepperoni, Provolone cheese, and green onions. Set aside or chill while making the dressing.

2. To make the dressing, add and mix the oil, vinegar, salt and pepper. Whisk the ingredients until the salt is fully dissolved. Pour salad dressing over the vegetables, toss to coat. Serve with grated Parmesan cheese on top.

Greek Chicken Souvlaki Salad

Marinated then grilled chicken skewers on top of a crunchy salad, and served with a refreshing yoghurt-cucumber dip. Perfect weekend fare.

SERVES: 4

INGREDIENTS:

FOR THE CHICKEN:

- ¼ cup of extra-virgin olive oil
- 2 tablespoons of fresh lemon juice
- 2 garlic cloves, minced
- 1 teaspoon of dried oregano
- ½ teaspoon of salt, to taste
- 2 pounds of chicken breast, deboned and skin removed, cut into cubes

FOR THE SAUCE:

- ¾ cups of Greek yogurt
- ½ cucumber, peeled and seeded, grated
- 2 tablespoons of extra-virgin olive oil

- 2 to 3 tablespoons white vinegar
- 1 garlic clove, minced
- A pinch of salt

FOR THE SALAD:

- 1 medium head of Red leaf lettuce, leaves separated
- ½ cup of Feta Cheese, crumbled
- 1 cup of Pepperoncini peppers, diced and seeded
- 1 cup of Kalamata Olives
- 1 cup cherry tomatoes, halved
- ½ medium cucumber, seeded and chopped
- 1 cup canned chickpeas, rinsed and drained

DIRECTIONS:

1. Cut the chicken into bite size pieces, place it on a plate and set aside.

2. In a resealable plastic, combine together lemon juice, garlic, oil, oregano and salt. Add in the chicken,

and make sure to remove air in the plastic. Refrigerate for at least two hours to marinate the meat.

3.   Preheat a grill pan or charcoal grill with high heat. Soak wooden skewers in water for 30 minutes prior to cooking.

4.   Place 5 to 7 pieces of marinated chicken pieces on each skewer. Cook the marinated chicken skewers in batches for 6 to 8 minutes per side, turning occasionally or until chicken is charred.

5.   In a mixing bowl, add and combine the yogurt, grated cucumber, olive oil, vinegar and garlic. Season with salt and extra dried herbs to taste.

6.   Portion lettuce leaves among 4 dinner plates. Top off with crumbled Feta cheese, olives, peppers, tomatoes, cucumbers and chickpeas. Place skewers on top of each plate, serve with salad dressing.

Baked Chicken Stuffed with Pesto and Cheese

Crispy chicken breast rolls with a cheesy creamy filling. Yay, I call this happy food!

SERVES: 2

INGREDIENTS:

- 2 chicken breasts, deboned and skin removed
- 2 tablespoons of lemon-basil pesto
- 2 tablespoons of sour cream, reduced fat
- 2 tablespoons of Mozzarella cheese, shredded
- 2 medium eggs, beaten
- 3 tablespoons of Parmesan cheese, finely grated
- 3 tablespoons of almond flour
- Freshly ground black pepper, as required
- Oil, for greasing

DIRECTIONS:

1. Preheat the stove to 375F. Lightly grease a small casserole using spray oil.

2. Trim excess lard from the chicken, now transfer each breast into a thick plastic bag, one at a time, pound each breast using a meat bat, so they become thin and even.

3. In a mixing bowl, combine together the sour cream, lemon-basil pesto, and shredded mozzarella cheese. Smear a layer of pesto-cream mixture with the use of a spatula covering both chicken breasts, leaving 1/2 inch clean around the chicken without the mixture. Enwrap the flattened chicken breast from the edge with the pesto-cream mixture to the other edge. Secure each chicken roll with toothpicks.

4. Take 2 bowls for breading the chicken rolls, one bowl containing the whisked egg, in the 2nd bowl add the Parmesan and flour mixed together with salt and pepper. Dip the chicken roll in the bowl with beaten egg. Next, dredge the breast rolls in the Parmesan and flour

mix, pat all sides of the breast rolls to make sure all areas are well-coated.

5. Place the chicken breasts in a greased casserole dish. Bake it in the oven for about 30 to 35 minutes, depending on the thickness of breast rolls. The breast rolls are done when it starts to turn brown to all sides. In order that the breast rolls will not be overcooked, check for doneness after 25 and 30 minutes in the oven.

6. Once the stuffed breast rolls are done, remove from the oven and let them stand for about 5 to 10 minutes. Serve whole or in round slices with leftover basil-pesto sauce.

Marsala Chicken and Mushroom Casserole

Good enough for lunch guests, but easy enough to make for the family.

SERVES: 2 to 4

INGREDIENTS:

- 2 tablespoons of unsalted butter

- 1 cup of mushrooms, halved

- 1 1/2 tablespoons of almond flour

- 1/2 cup of Marsala wine or any white wine

- 1/2 cup of heavy cream

- 2 tablespoons of fresh flat-leaf parsley, coarsely chopped

- Freshly ground black pepper and salt to taste

- 1 cup canned chickpeas, rinsed and drained

- 2 cups rotisserie chicken, cubed or cut into strips

- 2 tablespoons Parmesan cheese, grated

DIRECTIONS:

1. Preheat an oven to 350°F. Lightly grease a casserole dish with oil or butter. Set aside.

2. In a large non-stick skillet over medium –high heat, melt in the butter. Add the mushrooms and cook for about 4 to 5 minutes, stirring occasionally until soft. Dust the cooked mushrooms with flour on top, stir and cook for another 1 minute. Stir in the wine and cream, bring to a boil and cover with lid. Reduce heat to low and simmer for about 3 minutes, stirring occasionally until smooth and thick. Stir in 2 cups of water, chopped parsley leaves, season with salt and freshly ground black pepper to taste.

3. Spread an even layer of chickpea in a greased 9-inch-by-13-inch casserole, top with the chicken pieces. Pour over the mushroom gravy on top, Cover tightly with a foil and bake for about 35 minutes or until visible bubbles moves to the top surface. Remove and discard the foil, sprinkle with grated parmesan cheese on top. Return casserole in the oven, bake for 5 minutes in order

to brown and melt the cheese. Remove from the oven and let it stand for about 5 to 10 minutes before serving.

Low-Carb Tuscan Soup

Rich and aromatic, this soup will easily serve a crowd.

SERVES: 14

INGREDIENTS:

- 2 tablespoons of unsalted butter
- 2 cups of Turkey Italian Sausage, casing removed and sliced into thin rounds
- 6 cups of low-sodium beef broth
- 2 cups of kale, chopped
- 1 head of cauliflower, detached florets
- 6 cloves of garlic, minced
- 3 medium slices of bacon, sliced into small pieces
- 1 cup of heavy whipping cream

DIRECTIONS:

1. In a deep stock pot over medium-high heat, melt in the butter and brown sausage for about 5 to 7 minutes. Remove sausage from the pot then add the bacon and onion in the same pot. Cook until the onion is

soft and translucent, about 10 minutes and add the garlic. Cook for another 3 to 4 minutes, or until the garlic brown and aromatic.

2. Add 6 cups of beef broth and vegetables. Bring it to a steady boil for 35 minutes with lid on.

3. Remove pot from heat and stir in the heavy cream before serving. Add the sausage on top.

Crockpot Low-Carb Spicy Chicken Soup

Creamy and convenient, if you put this in the crockpot quickly after breakfast, it will be ready in time for lunch.

SERVES: 8

INGREDIENTS:

- 4 cups water
- 3 chicken breasts. Shredded
- 1/2 large onion, diced
- 1/4 head of cabbage, in chiffonades
- 1 cup tinned stewed tomatoes
- 1/2 cup of tinned red chillies
- 1 cup of salsa
- 1 cup cream cheese, softened
- 4 tablespoons heavy whipping cream
- 1 tablespoon garlic salt

- 1 tablespoon ground cumin
- Salt and black pepper, to taste

DIRECTIONS:

1. In the crock pot with 4 cups of water, place chicken breasts, onion and cabbage.
2. Cook for about 4 hours with high heat, or 6 to 8 hours on low until chicken is done. Take chicken out of the broth, cool and shred the meat into bite size pieces.
3. Return the chicken back in the pot, add the remaining ingredients and cook until cream cheese has melted and soup is thick and creamy.
4. Serve with sour cream on the side.

Low-Carb Avgolemono (Greek Chicken, Lemon & Egg Soup)

Fresh- tasting and light, this soup is also quick to make.

SERVES: 8

INGREDIENTS:

- 4 cups cooked, shredded chicken
- 10 cups chicken broth or stock
- 3 eggs
- 1/3 cup fresh lemon juice
- 2 cups cooked spaghetti squash
- 1/4 cup fresh parsley
- salt and pepper to taste
- 1 lemon, sliced into wedges
- freshly grated parmesan cheese (optional)

DIRECTIONS:

1. In a pot over high heat, add the broth and chicken breast. Bring it to a steady boil for 5 minutes, remove pot from heat.
2. In a mixing bowl, whisk the eggs and lemon juice until thick and frothy.
3. Gradually add in small amounts of 2 cups stock into the egg mixture, stirring constantly. Add the hot stock slowly and in gradual amounts to avoid cooking the eggs.
4. Once the chicken stock and the egg mixture are well incorporated, return the mixture in the pot.
5. Add in the spaghetti squash and season with salt and pepper to taste. Reheat the soup with low heat if needed and avoid the soup from boiling.
6. Serve warm with lemon wedges and fresh herbs on top.

Cream of Roasted Cauliflower Soup, with Cumin, Paprika, and Fresh Dill

This is a creamy, satisfying soup, with the flavours of hummus. If you don't have sumac, substitute some lemon zest instead.

SERVES: 5 to 6

INGREDIENTS:

- 2 medium heads of detached cauliflower florets
- 3 tablespoons of olive oil
- olive oil, for greasing
- Kosher salt, to taste
- Black pepper, to taste
- 1 small onion, diced
- 2 tablespoons of minced garlic
- ¼ to ½ of turmeric powder

- 1 to 2 teaspoons of sumac powder
- ½ tablespoon of cumin powder
- 2 ½ teaspoons Spanish paprika
- 4 to 5 cups of organic vegetable stock
- 1 cup water
- 2 to 2 ½ cups heavy cream
- 1 organic lemon, freshly juiced
- 1 cup fresh dill, coarsely chopped

DIRECTIONS:

1. Preheat the oven with a temperature of 425 °F. Lightly grease a baking sheet with oil, set aside.
2. Place the detached florets of cauliflower on the bottom of the greased baking sheet. Lightly brush with olive oil and dust with pepper and salt over the top.

3. Roast the vegetables for about 25 to 30 minutes, flipping over to cook the other side after the first 15 minutes. Remove vegetables from oven and let it rest

4. Meanwhile, heat 2 tablespoons olive oil in a large heavy pot or Dutch oven. In the heated oil, sauté onion until translucent. Add chopped garlic, cumin, turmeric, paprika and sumac. Stir together for a brief few seconds until fragrant.

5. Next add in ¾ of the roasted cauliflower, keep the rest for later. Stir to coat cauliflower well with the spices then add vegetable broth and water.

6. Bring to a simmer on medium-high heat. Cover and cook for five minutes or until cauliflower is aldenté as it takes in the liquid.

7. Uncover and remove from heat momentarily. Using and immersion blender, blend the cauliflower with the liquid until you reach a desired smoothness.

8. Return to a medium heat and stir in heavy cream with the lemon juice. Then add in the rest of roasted cauliflower florets you reserved earlier. Cook for a few minutes to warm the soup through. Test and add a pinch of salt if needed.

9. Finally, stir in the chopped dill.
10. Serve hot with your favorite bread.

LEPTIN MEDITERRANEAN HEALTHY DINNER RECIPES

In keeping with the leptin-friendly principle of having a light evening meal, and having it early, we've designed these recipes to be quick to make, and never heavy or too rich. We have some lovely seafood options, as well as vegetarian recipes for those meat-free Mondays, and also a beefy salad for when you crave a little red meat with your dinner.

Mediterranean Shrimp over Spinach

This is a quick weekday dinner, but much better than ordinary "fast food." Just be careful not to overcook the shrimp.

SERVES: 4

INGREDIENTS:

- 2 cups tinned diced tomatoes, drained
- 2 tablespoons of capers
- 2 cups of spinach leaves

- 1/2 large onion, diced
- 1 teaspoon garlic, finely minced
- 2 tablespoons olive oil, divided
- 1 large green bell pepper, deseeded and diced
- 1 teaspoon of Italian Herb Blend
- 1/2 cup fish stock
- salt and freshly ground black pepper, to taste
- 1 pound fresh large shrimp, shelled and deveined

DIRECTIONS:

1.	In a large pan over medium-high heat, add 1 tablespoon of olive oil. Once the oil is hot, sauté the onion and green bell pepper for about 3 to 4 minutes. Stir in the minced garlic and Italian herb, and then cook for another 2 minutes, stirring occasionally.

2.	Add the diced tomatoes and fish stock, cover lid and bring to a boil. Reduce to low heat and simmer for 10 minutes.

3.	In a separate pan, apply medium-high heat and add the oil. Once the oil is hot, add the spinach and cook for about 2 to 3 minutes, stirring occasionally. Remove pan from heat, set aside.

4. In the pan with sautéed vegetables, add the shrimp and capers. Cook for about 4 to 5 minutes or until the shrimp turns opaque in color. Season with salt and pepper to taste, cook for another minute.

5. Portion spinach into serving bowls and top with shrimp and capers. Serve hot.

Mediterranean Low-Carb "Cauliflower Risotto"

This is more foolproof than a traditional risotto, and eliminates the risk of gluey rice.

SERVES: 4

INGREDIENTS:

- 1 medium head cauliflower, detaches florets
- 2 tablespoons freshly chopped basil-oregano-thyme
- 2 tablespoons clarified butter
- ½ cup pesto sauce
- 2 cloves garlic, mashed
- 4 medium chicken breasts, skinned and deboned, diced
- ¼ cup heavy whipping cream or coconut milk
- ½ organic lemon, zested
- Pinch of freshly ground black pepper
- ½ teaspoon pink Himalayan or sea salt, to taste
- 1 cup Parmesan cheese, grated

DIRECTIONS:

1. Put the cauliflower florets in blender, pulse until you have a coarse texture to imitate the rice.
2. In a pan over medium-high heat, melt in the butter and add the diced chicken. Cook chicken for about 15 minutes, remove from pan. Transfer on a dish, set aside.
3. In the same pan over medium heat, melt in the remaining butter and cook lemon zest and garlic for about 3 to 4 minutes or until golden.
4. Add the cauliflower rice in the pan and cook for another 5 minutes, stirring constantly. Add the pesto sauce, cream and chopped herbs. Cook for another 2 to 3 minutes. Season to taste with salt and pepper.
5. Portion into serving plates, top off with grated Parmesan cheese. Serve warm.

Mediterranean Baked Fish, with Tomato-Onion-Garlic Sauce

Try this with any white fish. The delicious sauce keeps the fish from drying out in the oven.

SERVES: 4

INGREDIENTS:

- 1 teaspoon ground fennel seeds
- 1/2 teaspoon dried oregano
- 1 bay leaf
- 1 garlic clove, minced
- 3/4 cup of apple juice
- 1/2 cup tomato juice
- 1 1/2 teaspoon of dried thyme, crushed
- 1/2 teaspoon of dried basil, crushed
- 2 teaspoons olive oil extra virgin
- 1 Med - large onion, diced
- 2 cups canned whole tomatoes, drained and diced
- 4 cups of lemon juice
- 1/4 cup of orange juice

- 1 tablespoon freshly grated orange peel
- black pepper, to taste
- 1 pound flounder fillets

DIRECTIONS:

1. In a skillet, apply medium heat and add the oil. Once the oil is hot, sauté the onions for about 4 minutes or until soft and translucent.

2. Stir in all of the remaining ingredients except for the fish. Stir it thoroughly, cover with a lid and simmer for about 30 minutes.

3. Preheat an oven to 350°F.

4. Grease a baking dish and add the fish fillets. Pour over the sauce to cover.

5. Bake in the oven for about 15 minutes or until the fish easily flakes.

Shrimp Saganaki

Saganaki is a Greek appetizer, made with a thick slice of cheese, dusted with flour and then fried till the middle is melted. It gets its name from the small two-handled heavy frying pan in which it's made. It's basically a chunk of fried cheese for a meze platter, but in this version it's made into a complete meal with the addition of shrimp and some vegetables.

SERVES: 4

INGREDIENTS:

- 12 large shrimp, deveined and peeled
- 1/2 cup Chardonnay wine
- 1/2 cup Feta cheese, crumbled
- 1 tablespoon of extra-virgin olive oil
- 1 medium fennel bulb, cored and finely diced
- 2 tablespoons lemon juice, divided
- 1/4 teaspoon salt
- 5 scallions, finely cut
- 1 chilli pepper, such as jalapeño or Serrano, seeded and minced
- Ground black pepper, to taste

DIRECTIONS:

1. In a bowl, add shrimp, salt and lemon juice. Toss and set aside.
2. In a skillet, apply medium heat and add the oil. Once the oil is hot, add scallions, fennel and chilli pepper. Cook for about 4 to 5 minutes, stirring constantly until soft. Add in the wine, cook for another minute and add the shrimp on top of the sautéed ingredients. Cook with lid on, for about 4 minutes. Remove skillet from heat.
3. Transfer the shrimp on a serving dish. Add the remaining lemon juice, pepper and Feta in the skillet and cook until the cheese is melted.
4. Transfer the vegetables on a serving dish and top off with shrimp. Serve warm.

Grilled Shrimp Salad with Feta, Tomato, and Watermelon

This pretty salad combines all the colors of the Italian flag, and then gets topped with delicious flame-grilled shrimp skewers.

SERVES: 4

INGREDIENTS:

- 1/4 cup extra-virgin olive oil
- 1-1/2 teaspoon of local honey
- Vegetable oil, for the grill
- 1 1/2 pound large fresh shrimp, peeled and deveined
- 1/4 cup and 2 tablespoon fresh lemon juice
- 1 teaspoon paprika
- salt and freshly cracked black pepper, to taste
- 1/2 medium head of frisée, torn into small pieces
- 3 cups watermelon, deseeded and diced
- 3 red tomatoes, cut into wedges
- 2 cups cherry tomatoes, cut into halves

- ¾ cup Feta cheese, diced
- 1/2 cup fresh basil leaves, shredded

DIRECTIONS:

1. Prepare a gas or charcoal grill, and preheat with high heat.
2. Mix lemon juice and paprika in a mixing bowl, stir in the shrimp. Toss to coat, set aside and marinate for about 5 minutes. Season shrimp with salt and pepper, thread into skewers.
3. Mix together ¼ cup lemon juice, honey, oil, and a pinch of pepper and salt. Mix it thoroughly, set aside.
4. Scrape off the burnt food in the cooking grates and brush with oil. Grill the skewered shrimps, flipping occasionally to cook them evenly. Cook for about 5 to 6 minutes in total, or until opaque and firm.
5. In a mixing bowl, toss in the tomatoes, basil, cheese, watermelon, 2 tablespoon of dressing, salt and pepper. In a separate mixing bowl, toss frisée with 3 tablespoons of dressing and portion into serving bowls. Portion into each serving bowl the watermelon-tomato

mixture and top off with shrimp skewers. Drizzle with the remaining dressing on top, serve.

Orecchiette with Mussels & Mint

This dish packs big flavour with just a few ingredients. It's quick to make, too.

SERVES: 4

INGREDIENTS:

- 1 tablespoon of salt
- 2 medium zucchini, cut into batonnets
- 1/2 cup heavy cream
- 1 recipe of orecchiette
- A dozen of mussels, cleaned
- 1/2 cup dry white wine
- Salt and freshly ground black pepper, to taste
- 1/4 cup fresh mint leaves, chopped

DIRECTIONS:

1. Add water in a pot over high heat, bring to a boil and add salt and orecchiette. Cook for about 8 minutes or until done.

2.	In a frying pan, add the mussels and wine, apply medium heat and cover. Bring to a boil and cook for about 2 to 3 minutes, or until the mussels have opened. Remove the mussels with a slotted spoon, strain the mussel stock with cheesecloth and return in the pan. Add the zucchini, return to a boil and simmer for about 3 minutes or until soft.

3.	Remove the shells of the mussels, discard shells and add the meat in the pan with the zucchini.
 Stir in the cream, season with salt and pepper.

4.	Toss the orecchiette into the pan, cook until the sauce starts to thicken, or for about 2 minutes. Top off with mint, serve.

Greek-Style Shrimp Salad

A lovely light dinner dish, where the tang of olives and capers are balanced with the creaminess of the cheese.

SERVES: 4

INGREDIENTS:

- 1 pound of fresh, large shrimps, peeled and deveined
- 1/4 cup pitted black olives, chopped
- 1 tablespoon capers, drained and rinsed
- 5 tablespoons of extra-virgin olive oil
- 1 teaspoon dried oregano
- salt and coarsely ground black pepper, to taste
- 1 cup plum tomatoes, diced and seeded
- ½ cup Feta cheese or goat's cheese, crumbled
- 1 tablespoon red wine vinegar
- 1 tablespoon fresh lemon juice, organic
- 1 cup baby greens, washed and drained

DIRECTIONS:

1. Preheat a broiler to high and place an oven rack on top rung.
2. Mix together the oil, salt and pepper in a bowl and toss in the shrimp. Cover a baking sheet with foil and layer the shrimp on it. Broil the shrimp for about 5 minutes, or until opaque inside and pink on the outside.
3. While broiling the shrimp, combine capers, lemon juice, feta, olives, tomatoes, oregano, oil, vinegar and the remaining lemon juice in a mixing bowl. When the shrimp is done, toss it with tomato-feta mixture.
4. Add the greens, toss to combine and portion into individual serving bowls. Serve with extra herbs and cheese on top.

Halibut and Mussel Stew with Fennel, Peppers, and Saffron

Use the crunchy garlic toasts to mop up all the delicious juices.

SERVES: 4

INGREDIENTS:

- 2 tablespoons olive oil, extra-virgin
- 1 yellow onion, sliced thinly
- 1 fennel bulb, trimmed and quartered
- salt and freshly ground black pepper, to taste
- 4 baguette slices, 1 inch thick
- 2 to 3 tablespoons of tomato paste
- 2 cloves of garlic, crushed
- 1/2 cup dry white wine (Albariño)
- 1 carrot, peeled and sliced thinly
- 1 ½ cup of halibut fillets, cut into bite size pieces
- 1 dozen of fresh mussels, cleaned
- 2 pinches of saffron
- 1 bay leaf

- 1 red bell pepper, seeded and sliced into strips
- 1 cup canned chickpeas, drained and rinsed
- 1 teaspoon fresh thyme leaves, minced
- A pinch of pimento

DIRECTIONS:

1. In a saucepan with oil over medium heat, add the onion, fennel, carrot, and bell pepper. Cook for about 5 to 6 minutes, stirring it until the vegetables are tender.

2. Stir in the tomato paste and garlic in the saucepan, cook for about 1 minute. Stir constantly and add in the wine. Cover lid and bring to a simmer, cook until thickened and reduced by half. Add 3 cups of water, chickpeas, bay leaf, thyme, pimenton and saffron. Bring to a boil and cover, cook for about 20 to 25 minutes or vegetables are tender and sauce has thickened. Season with salt and black pepper to taste.

3. Preheat the broiler on high, place the bread slices brushed with oil on a baking sheet. Broil for about 2 minutes on each side, flipping once to cook the other side until golden-brown.

4. Remove bread from the oven and rub with crushed garlic, place it on a serving dish.

5. Add the halibut and mussels into the pan with the stew, cover and simmer for about 4 to 8 minutes, or until the fish is cooked and all the mussels have opened.

6. Ladle stew into shallow bowls, serve with the garlic toasts.

Tilapia Feta Florentine

A richly satisfying bake, full of nutritious goodness.

SERVES: 4

INGREDIENTS:

- 1 garlic clove, minced
- 2 cups of fresh spinach, chopped
- 1/4 cup olives, sliced
- 1 tablespoon of olive oil
- 1/4 cup onion, diced
- ½ teaspoon of dried oregano
- ½ teaspoon of white pepper
- 2 tablespoons Feta cheese or goat's cheese, crumbled
- 1/2 teaspoon zest lemon rind
- 1/2 teaspoon salt, to taste
- 3 to 4 tilapia fillets
- 2 tablespoons of unsalted butter, melted
- 2 teaspoons of fresh lemon juice
- 1 pinch paprika, to taste

DIRECTIONS:

1. Preheat an oven to 400°F. Grease a 9x13 baking dish, set aside.
2. In a skillet over medium-high heat, heat the oil. Once the oil is hot, sauté the garlic and onion for about 4 minutes, or until soft and fragrant. Stir in the spinach and cook for 4 minutes until wilted. Add in the lemon zest, oregano, pepper, olives, cheese and salt to the skillet. Cook for another 4 minutes or until the cheese has melted.
3. Lay the spinach on the greased baking dish and place tilapia on top. Drizzle with butter-lemon mixture and sprinkle with smoked paprika.

Bake it in oven for 20 to 25 minutes, or until the fish is flaky and cooked through.

Gyro Salad

A delicious green salad topped with strips of seasoned beef.

SERVES: 4

INGREDIENTS:

YOGURT DRESSING:

- ½ cup Greek yogurt
- ½ cup reduced-fat sour cream
- ¼ cup milk
- 1 teaspoon of Greek seasoning

SALAD:

- 1 sirloin steak beef or about 1 pound, cut into strips
- 1 tablespoon of extra virgin olive oil
- 2 teaspoons of Greek seasoning
- 8 cups of mixed salad greens
- 1 medium cucumber, seeded and thinly sliced
- 1 red onion, sliced into thin rounds

- 1 large ripe tomato, diced

DIRECTIONS:

1. In a mixing bowl, whisk together all of the dressing ingredients until smooth and creamy.
2. In a skillet over medium-high heat, add the oil. Once the oil is hot, add the beef and the Greek seasoning. Cook until beef is brown, stirring frequently for about 5 to 7 minutes. Drain if necessary.
3. Portion salad greens on serving plates and top off with cucumber, onion, tomato and strips of beef. Serve with dressing on top.

LEPTIN MEDITERRANEAN HEALTHY SOUP RECIPES

Soup is a great option for a light dinner, or for those times when you're feeling peckish but want a healthy snack. It's the ultimate fast food too, as many soups can be cooked within half an hour. Preparation is usually done in one pot, leaving you with less washing up to do!

Many of the soups in this chapter will freeze well, so you could make a batch and freeze single portions for convenience.

Cabbage Soup with Kielbasa

Kielbasa is a type of smoked sausage, which pairs perfectly with cabbage in this soup which is bursting both with flavour and goodness.

SERVES: 4

INGREDIENTS:

- 2 cups of Kielbasa, sliced into thin rounds
- 2 cups of cabbage, cut into chiffonades
- 2 medium zucchini, sliced into rounds

- 2 green pepper, diced
- 2 tablespoon extra-virgin olive oil
- 2 small yellow pepper, diced
- 1 medium onion, diced
- 2 cups of tomato juice
- 1 cup of canned stewed tomatoes
- 2 cups vegetable stock
- 1 tablespoon red hot chilli powder
- ½ teaspoon of ground black pepper
- ½ teaspoon salt
- 1 medium stalk celery , chopped
- ½ cup of fresh mushrooms, quartered

•

DIRECTIONS:

1. In a pan, apply medium-high heat and add 1 tablespoon of oil. Once the oil is hot, add the onion, diced peppers, and celery. Cook for about 5 minutes until soft and tender. Stir in the mushrooms and cook for another 3 minutes. Remove pan from heat, set aside.

In a separate pan, apply medium-high heat and add the oil. Add in sliced Kielbasa and cook for about 4 to 5 minutes. Stir in the sautéed vegetables and cook for 2 to 3 minutes, stirring occasionally. Add in the stewed tomatoes, tomato juice, chilli powder and season with the seasoning. Heat to a boil, then turn the heat to low and simmer for 5 minutes, stirring occasionally. Remove from heat, set aside.

2. In a large saucepan, pour in the vegetable stock and heat to a boil. Blanche the zucchini in the boiling stock for about 2 to 3 minutes, remove from pot and transfer into a bowl with ice bath. Drain zucchini and set aside. Blanche the cabbage for about 2 minutes in the pot, remove from pot and place into a bowl with ice bath. Drain and set aside.

3. In the pot, stir in the simmered ingredients from the pan and bring to a boil. Add the blanched vegetables and return to a boil. Remove pot from heat, portion soup into serving bowls. Serve warm.

Chilled Red Pepper Soup with Sautéed Shrimp

Serve this refreshing soup in the summer months, when a hot dinner is just not what you feel like.

SERVES: 6

INGREDIENTS:

- 1 cup croutons
- 2 garlic cloves, mashed into paste
- 1 cucumber, peeled and deseeded, chopped
- 1 lemon, sliced into wedges
- ½ cup canned/jarred roasted red peppers, diced
- 2 cups tomato juice
- 1/2 teaspoon ground cumin
- 4 tablespoons extra-virgin olive oil
- 3 tablespoons cider vinegar
- Salt and coarsely ground black pepper

- 2 dozen small shrimps, peeled and deveined
- 1 tablespoon fresh thyme leaves, minced
- ½ cup fish stock

DIRECTIONS:

1. In a food processor or blender, add the cucumber, red pepper, tomato juice, croutons, 4 tablespoons of oil and 2 tablespoons of vinegar. Add ½ cup fish stock and pulse until smooth, season with cumin, salt and pepper and pulse again until you have a thick and smooth mixture. Transfer into a bowl, cover and chill in the fridge.

2. In a pan, apply medium-high heat and add the remaining oil. Once the oil is hot, add the garlic paste and shrimp. Cook for 5 minutes, stirring occasionally. Season with salt and pepper to taste. Cool and chill in the refrigerator.

3. Remove the chilled soup and portion into individual serving bowls. Top off with minced thyme and peeled shrimp, and serve with lemon wedges.

Grilled Watermelon Gazpacho with Lime Cream

A very refreshing chilled soup, perfect for a summer evening.

SERVES: 5

INGREDIENTS:

- 2 medium tomatoes, diced
- 2 medium cucumber, peeled and cubed
- 2 tablespoons extra-virgin olive oil
- 1 Serrano chilli, deseeded and diced
- 1 organic lime, juiced
- 1 teaspoons chipotle chilli powder
- 1 medium watermelon, sliced into wedges
- Kosher salt, to taste
- 1/4 cup fresh cilantro, minced
- 1 shallot, minced
- 1 to 2 tablespoons red wine vinegar
- 1/4 cup crème fraîche

DIRECTIONS:

1. Prepare a charcoal or gas grill set up, preheat to high.
2. In a small bowl, combine 1 tablespoon of oil, salt and chipotle. Lightly brush the watermelon with the mixture. Grill for about 2 minutes on each side, or until nicely charred. Remove from grill and set aside to cool. Remove the rinds and seeds, and dice the flesh.
3. In a food processor, add the watermelon, tomato, cilantro, shallot, cucumber, chilli and the remaining oil. Pulse for 1 minute and add half of the lime juice and vinegar. Pulse again until you have a smooth and thick mixture. Season with salt and pepper, place in a bowl and chill for at least 2 hours.
4. Before serving, combine crème fraîche and the remaining lime juice in a bowl. Portion soup into individual serving bowls, drizzle with cream-lime mixture on top.

White Gazpacho with Grapes and Toasted Almonds

Gazpacho is a cold soup, with Spanish origins.

SERVES: 4

INGREDIENTS:

- 3 slices of white bread, edges trimmed, soaked
- ¼ cup almonds
- 2 medium cucumbers, deseeded and diced
- 1/2 cup of warm water
- 3 cloves garlic, peeled and crushed
- 1 tablespoon of fresh organic lemon juice, or as needed to taste
- 5 scallions, green parts trimmed off and thinly sliced
- 1/4 cup sherry vinegar, or as needed to taste
- 1/2 teaspoon of salt, or as needed to taste
- 3 tablespoons of extra-virgin olive oil
- ½ cup green grapes, halved

DIRECTIONS:

1. In a pan, apply medium-high heat and toast the almonds in. Cook for 4 to 5 minutes until browned and fragrant, tossing occasionally. Remove from pan, set aside.

2. Reserve ¼ of cucumber, 1 tablespoon almonds, and 1 tablespoon of scallion for garnish, set aside. In a food processor, add the remaining cucumber, crushed garlic, soaked bread, scallions, vinegar, lemon juice, almonds, salt and oil. Pulse until you have a uniform-sized mixture of ingredients and add more salt and vinegar, if needed. Pulse again until a smooth and thick mixture is achieved.

3. Portion into individual serving bowls, serve with cucumber, scallions, grapes and toasted almonds on top.

Mediterranean Kale & White Bean Soup with Sausage

SERVES: 6 to 8

INGREDIENTS:

- 3 links of sweet Italian sausage, casings removed and chopped
- Salt and coarsely ground black pepper
- 5 cups chicken broth
- 1 carrot, peeled and diced
- 1 celery stalk, cut into small dice
- ½ pound kale, stems removed and leaves coarsely chopped
- 2 tablespoons of fresh organic lemon juice
- 2 tablespoons of olive oil
- Pinch of red pepper flakes, crushed
- 2 cups of cooked dried beans
- 1 small yellow onion, diced
- 4 garlic cloves, minced
- 1/2 teaspoon zest of lemon

DIRECTIONS:

1. Heat 1 tablespoon of oil in a large saucepan and place on a medium-high heat. Put in the sausage and fry for about 4 minutes, occasionally stir. Remove from pot, transfer into a plate and leave the oil.
2. Add the remaining oil in the pot. Add the onion and cook for about 2 minutes, stirring occasionally. Stir in the carrot and celery, cook for another 2 minutes until browned and tender. Stir in the garlic, pepper flakes, ground black pepper and salt in the pot. Cook for 2 minutes until the garlic is fragrant, add the broth and reduce heat to high.
3. Add the sausage and half of the beans, mash remaining beans and add into the pot. Cover lid and bring to a boil. When it starts to boil, add the kale and reduce heat to low and simmer for 15 minutes. Add the lemon zest and juice, adjust seasoning to desired taste.
4. Remove pot from heat and portion soup into individual serving bowls. Serve warm.

Moroccan Vegetable Ragoût

A ragoût is a traditional French stew, and the name literally means "to revive the taste." This lovely vegetarian option will certainly revive your taste buds, as well as deliver a good dose of vitamins at the same time

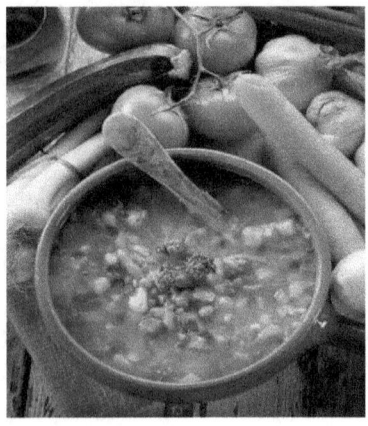

SERVES: 3 to 4

INGREDIENTS:

- 1 tablespoon olive oil, extra-virgin
- 1 orange, juiced
- 2 teaspoons of local honey

- 1 yellow onion, thinly sliced
- 2 cups sweet potatoes, peeled and diced
- 2 cups canned chickpeas, drained and rinsed
- 1 cup canned diced tomatoes
- 1 cinnamon stick
- 1 cup vegetable stock
- 2 teaspoons ground cumin
- ½ cup green Greek or Italian olives, pitted
- 2 cups kale leaves, lightly packed and chopped
- Kosher salt and roughly ground black pepper, to taste

DIRECTIONS:

1. In a pot over medium-high heat, add the oil. When hot, put in the onion and cook for about 4 minutes until soft and translucent. Add cinnamon stick, cumin, potatoes, tomatoes, chickpeas, olives, orange juice, honey and stock in the pot. Cover lid and bring to a boil.

2. Once it starts to boil, reduce to low heat and simmer for 15 minutes. Add in the kale and give it a quick stir and cover. Simmer for another 10 minutes, or

Up to the vegetables are soft and tender. Season with salt and black pepper to taste.

3. Remove pot from heat, portion soup into serving bowls and serve warm.

Cucumber-Yogurt Soup with Avocado

Another chilled soup: pretty, light, and packed full of vitamins.

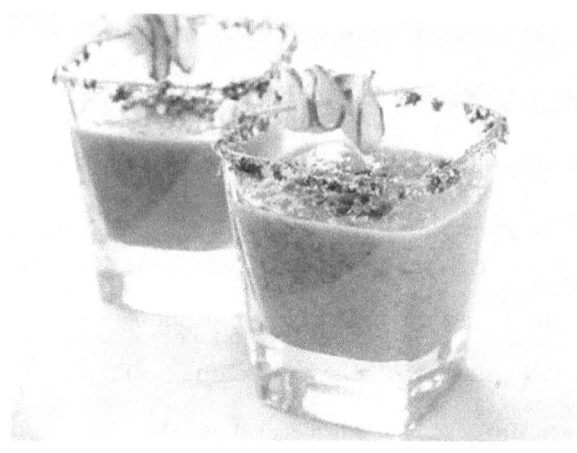

SERVES: 4

INGREDIENTS:

- 2 tablespoons extra-virgin olive oil

- 1 teaspoon garlic, minced
- 2 medium cucumbers, peeled and seeded, diced
- 1 medium ripe avocado, peeled and pitted, diced
- 1 cup plain yogurt
- 1 teaspoon toasted cumin seeds, ground
- 1 teaspoon salt, or as needed to taste
- 1 large white onion, diced
- 2 tablespoons minced fresh basil leaves
- 2 tablespoons minced fresh mint leaves
- 3 tablespoons fresh lemon juice
- Coarsely ground black pepper, as needed to taste

DIRECTIONS:

1. Add the onion and cucumber in a food processor, pulse until a coarse mixture is achieved. Take out ½ cup of the onion-cucumber mixture, place it in a bowl and set aside.
2. Add the avocado in the processor, together with oil, yogurt, garlic and season with cumin and salt. Purée the ingredients until a smooth consistency is achieved.
3. Place the puréed ingredients in a bowl, stir in the basil, mint, lemon juice, remaining onion-cucumber mixture and ½ cup of water. Stir to combine, adjust consistency by adding more water and then season with salt and pepper. Cover and chill for at least 1 hour before serving.
4. Portion chilled soup into individual serving bowls. Serve.

Roasted Red Pepper & Tomato Gazpacho

While the cheese at the end is optional, it does add a lovely contrast in texture, flavour, and color.

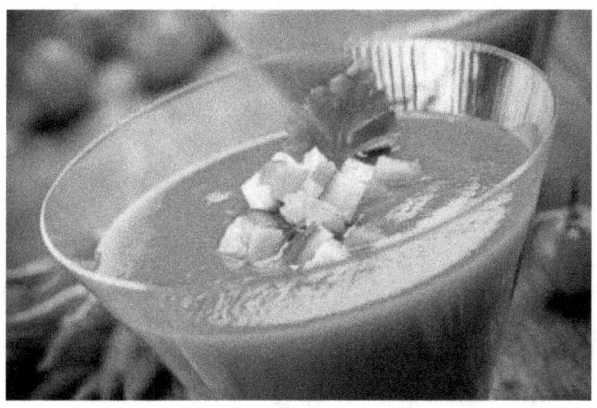

SERVES: 4

INGREDIENTS:

- 2 red bell peppers, seeded and halved
- 3 cups of ripe tomatoes, seeded and diced
- 3 garlic cloves, minced
- 4 tablespoons extra-virgin olive oil, or as needed
- 1 organic lemon, juiced
- 4 scallions, chopped

- 2 cucumbers, peeled and seeded, diced
- 1/2 cup mixed fresh herbs, chopped (thyme, chervil, basil, parsley, marjoram, and tarragon)
- salt and coarsely ground black pepper, to taste
- 1/4 cup goat's cheese, crumbled (optional)

DIRECTIONS:

1. Roast the peppers in a preheated broiler for about 10 minutes, or until the skin is nicely charred. Transfer into a covered container, set aside to cool. Peel off the skin from the roasted peppers.

2. Put the roasted peppers and tomatoes in a food processor, pulse into a mixture with coarse texture.

3. Transfer into a large bowl, stir in the garlic and gradually add in the oil while constantly stirring. Add in the lemon juice, cucumber, scallions and half of the chopped herb mixture and stir to combine.

4. Chill for at least an hour before serving. Portion chilled soup into individual serving bowls, top with crumbled cheese and herb mixture. Drizzle with olive oil and serve.

Lemony Egg Soup with Peas

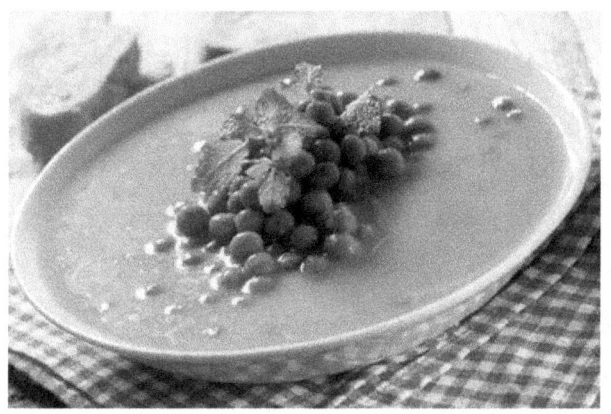

SERVES: 4 to 6

INGREDIENTS:

- 2 tablespoons of unsalted butter
- 1 shallot, minced
- 1 cup chicken broth
- 1 lemon, juiced
- 2 large eggs
- salt and coarsely ground black pepper
- 2 tablespoons of Parmigiano-Reggiano, grated
- 2 cups cooked peas

DIRECTIONS:

1. Melt the butter in pot over medium heat. Add the shallots and cook for about 2 minutes, or until soft and translucent. Add the broth and lemon juice, cover and bring to a boil. Reduce to low heat and simmer for 10 minutes.

2. While cooking the soup, add and whisk together the eggs, salt and pepper. Gradually pour small amounts of the egg mixture in the pot, stirring constantly. Add the cheese, season with salt and pepper. Return to a simmer, remove pot from heat.

3. Portion into individual serving bowls, serve with cooked peas on top.

Mediterranean Roasted Vegetable Soup

Roasting the vegetables first brings out all their delicious sweetness. Pumpkin seeds make a lovely garnish, echoing the butternut squash in the soup.

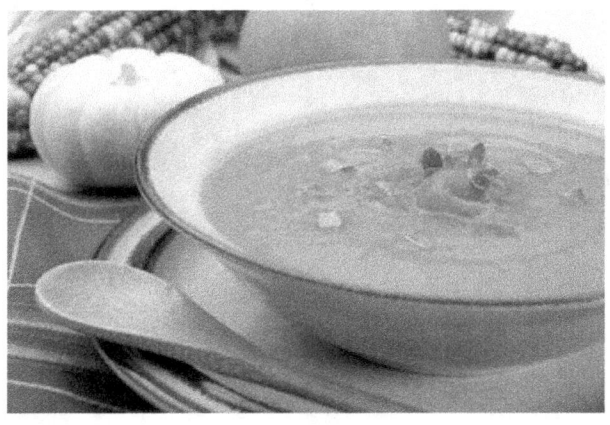

SERVES: 6

INGREDIENTS:

- 1 yellow pepper, deseeded and sliced into strips
- 1 large red onion, cut into wedges
- 1 small butternut squash, peeled and divided into 8 equal portions
- 1 red pepper, sliced into strips

- 2 large tomatoes, cut into quarters
- 1 tablespoon minced garlic
- 3 sprigs rosemary
- 1 organic lemon, juiced
- salt and freshly ground black pepper, to taste
- 2 cups vegetable stock

DIRECTIONS:

1.	Preheat oven to 200°C. Grease a roasting tin with oil, set aside.
2.	Place the vegetable on the greased roasting tin. Top with garlic, rosemary, salt and pepper, and then drizzle with lemon juice on top.
3.	Roast in the oven for about 30 minutes, or until the vegetables are tender and cooked through. Discard the rosemary, set aside to cool.
4.	Place half of the vegetables and the stock in a food processor. Pulse until a smooth and thick consistency is achieved.
5.	Portion the remaining roasted vegetables into individual serving bowls. Reheat the pureed vegetables and pour into serving bowls. Serve warm.

LEPTIN MEDITERRANEAN HEALTHY SALAD RECIPES

There's so much more to salads than boring old iceberg lettuce and tomatoes. Use these unusual salads as side dishes, or as a light meal, perhaps accompanied by a lovely crispy crusted loaf.

Mediterranean Cucumber & Tomato Salad

SERVES: 6 to 8

INGREDIENTS:

- 2 medium cucumbers, diced
- 3 large tomatoes, diced
- 1 onion, diced or thinly sliced
- 2 tablespoons minced fresh basil
- 2 tablespoons minced fresh cilantro
- 2 tablespoons minced fresh parsley
- Salt and black pepper, to taste
- 1 organic lemon, juiced
- 4 tablespoons extra virgin olive oil

DIRECTIONS:

1. Mix together the cucumber, tomato, onion and minced herbs in a bowl. Season with salt and pepper to taste. Gently toss the ingredients to combine.
2. Cover and chill for at least 2 hours before serving.
3. Remove the bowl from the chiller and stir in the lemon juice and olive oil. Briefly toss the salad to combine.
4. Portion salad into serving bowls then serve.

Feta Salad with Pomegranate Dressing

This salad contains the "Fruit of Paradise" as pomegranates are sometimes known. They're sweet, crunchy, and brimming with antioxidants.

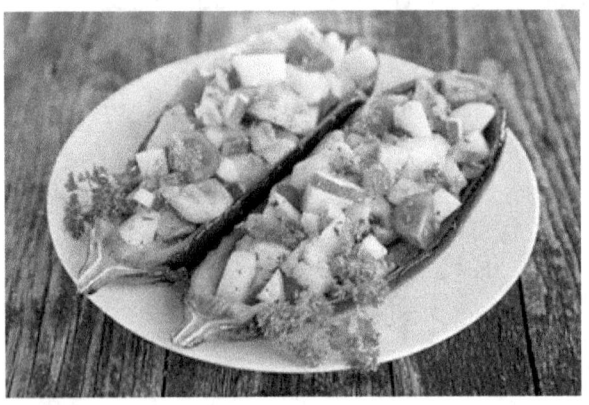

SERVES: 8

INGREDIENTS:

- 2 red bell peppers, seeded and halved/ quartered
- 3 medium aubergines, halved/quartered
- ¼ cup extra virgin olive oil
- 1 teaspoon cinnamon
- 1 cup chickpeas, blanched
- 1 red onion, halved and thinly sliced

- 1 cup feta cheese, crumbled
- ¼ cup of pomegranate seeds
- ¼ cup of fresh parsley, roughly chopped

FOR THE DRESSING:

- 2 garlic clove, minced
- 1 tablespoon lemon juice
- 2 tablespoons pomegranate molasses
- 4 tablespoons extra virgin olive oil

DIRECTIONS:

1. Preheat oven to 200°C. Place the peppers skin side up, on a greased baking sheet. On a separate greased baking sheet, place the aubergines and drizzle with olive oil. Season with cinnamon, salt and pepper.

2. Roast the peppers and the aubergines at the same time in the oven. Roast peppers for about 5 minutes, or until blackened. Transfer roasted peppers to a resealable plastic bag, set aside to cool. Scrape off the skin of the roasted peppers, discard the skin and set aside the peppers.

3.   Roast aubergines for about 20 to 25 minutes until softened. Remove from the oven, set aside.

4.   While roasting the vegetables, combine all ingredients for the dressing in a mixing bowl. Whisk to combine, set aside.

5.   Portion aubergines into serving plates together with the greens, onions, and roasted peppers. Pour the dressing over and top with parsley. Serve.

Fig & Mozzarella salad

Just reading this recipe makes my mouth water. The combination of honey-sweet figs, crunchy hazelnuts and beans, and creamy cheese is simply stunning.

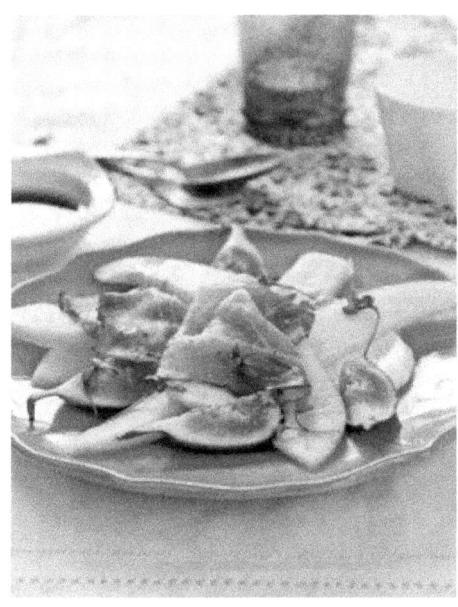

SERVES: 4

INGREDIENTS:

- 200g fine green beans, trimmed and blanched
- ½ cup fresh basil leaves, torn

- 2 tablespoons balsamic vinegar
- 6 small figs, quartered
- 1 shallot, thinly sliced
- 1 ball mozzarella, drained and diced
- ¼ cup hazelnuts, toasted and chopped
- 1 ½ tablespoons fig jam
- Salt and pepper, to taste
- 3 tablespoons extra-virgin olive oil

DIRECTIONS:

1. Portion blanched beans on individual serving plates, top off with shallots, figs, hazelnuts and basil.
2. Combine together fig jam, olive oil, balsamic vinegar in a bowl, season with salt and pepper. Whisk to combine.
3. Pour the dressing over the salad mixture and serve with cheese and extra basil on top.

Shredded Romaine and Cucumber Salad with Yogurt Dressing

This fresh green salad has a lot of flavour and looks so pretty on the plate.

SERVES: 4

INGREDIENTS:

FOR THE DRESSING:

- 2 garlic cloves, minced
- 1/2 cup Greek yogurt
- ½ organic fresh lemon, juiced
- 1 tablespoon white vinegar
- 1 to 2 teaspoons sugar
- 5 tablespoons extra-virgin olive oil
- salt and ground black pepper

FOR THE SALAD:

- 1 tablespoon chopped fresh mint
- 2 tablespoons chopped fresh flat-leaf parsley

- 1 cup of baby arugula, chopped
- ½ cup toasted walnut halves, chopped
- 2 tablespoons chopped fresh dill
- 1 large head of romaine lettuce, cut into chiffonades
- 1 cucumber, seeded and thinly sliced
- salt and ground black pepper, to taste
- ½ teaspoon red pepper flakes, crushed

DIRECTIONS:

1. In a mixing bowl, combine together the lemon juice, sugar, garlic and vinegar. Let it stand for at least 5 minutes to infuse the flavors. Whisk in the yogurt and gradually drizzle in the oil, whisking constantly to combine the ingredients. Season to taste with salt and ground pepper. Chill until ready to use.

2. Pat dry the romaine leaves with paper towels and transfer to a large bowl. Mix in the cucumbers, walnuts, dill, mint and parsley in the bowl. Chill for at least 1 hour before serving.

3. Remove the salad mixture from the chiller and toss it with the dressing. Serve with red pepper flakes and extra walnuts on top.

Shaved Fennel Salad with Toasted Almonds, Lemon, and Mint

Combining typically Mediterranean ingredients, this is another simple but beautiful dish.

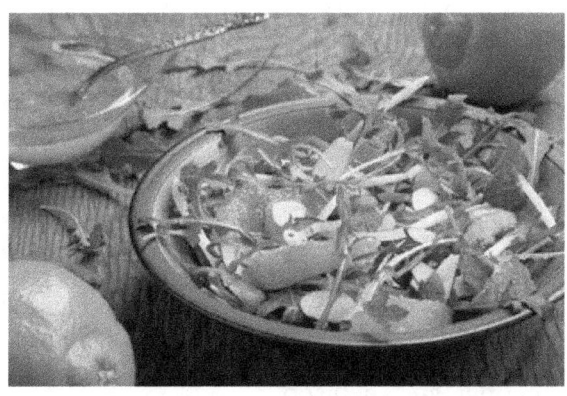

SERVES: 4 to 6

INGREDIENTS:

- 1/4 cup fresh mint leaves, torn
- 1/4 cup extra-virgin olive oil
- ½ teaspoon of coarsely ground black pepper
- 2 large fennel bulbs, trimmed and core removed
- 1 organic lemon/orange, juiced
- Kosher salt, to taste

- 1/2 cup chopped almonds, toasted

DIRECTIONS:

1. Shave the fennel crosswise with a mandolin. Place in a bowl, set aside.
2. In the bowl, toss fennel with lemon juice and salt. Let it stand for 10 minutes to infuse the flavors. Stir in half the almonds, mint and the olive oil, toss to combine.
3. Portion salad into individual serving plates. Top with the remaining almonds and mint, finish off with freshly cracked pepper, and then serve.

Brooklyn Grange Salad with Pickled Eggs and Idiazabal

Idiazabal is a traditional hard cheese made from raw sheep's milk, and originating in Spain.

SERVES: 6

INGREDIENTS:

- 1/2 cup toasted honey pecans
- 2 cups grated radish
- 1 medium kohlrabi, grated thinly with mandolin
- 1 garlic clove, crushed
- salt and ground black pepper, to taste
- 3 tablespoons sherry vinegar
- 1 teaspoon red pepper flakes, crushed
- 2 tablespoons minced anchovy fillets
- sea salt
- ½ cup finely grated Idiazabal or Manchego cheese
- 1 tablespoon preserved lemons, finely chopped
- ¼ cup of olive oil
- 1 tablespoons Dijon mustard
- 4 cups of baby greens, roughly chopped

- 1 cup mixed fresh herbs and edible flowers, herbs cut into chiffonades
- ½ tablespoon of finely grated organic lemon zest

FOR THE PICKLED EGGS:

- 5 to 6 eggs, soft boiled and shells removed

- 1 cup pickled beets, solids and liquid separated

DIRECTIONS:

1. Place the eggs in a non-reactive container and pour pickling liquid to cover. Cover the container and chill for at least one day.
2. Put 2 teaspoons of oil, garlic, lemons, anchovies, teaspoon of salt and pepper in a mortar. Grind the mixture into a paste with a pestle. Transfer the paste to a mixing bowl and mix in the vinegar and mustard. Gradually stir in the oil, season with salt and pepper. Set aside.

3. In a separate bowl, add in the radishes, kohlrabi, pecans, greens, chopped herbs and mixed flowers. Adjust taste with pepper and salt. Gently toss ingredients with vinaigrette, place into a serving dish. Set aside.

4. Remove eggs and transfer into a colander, drain liquid and pat dry with paper towels. Slice the eggs into halves and place it over the salad mixture. Top with cheese, horseradish and grated zest of lemon, serve.

Poached Quince Salad

Quinces lend a lovely sweetness to this salad, and contrast well with the bitterness of the arugula and the saltiness of the ham.

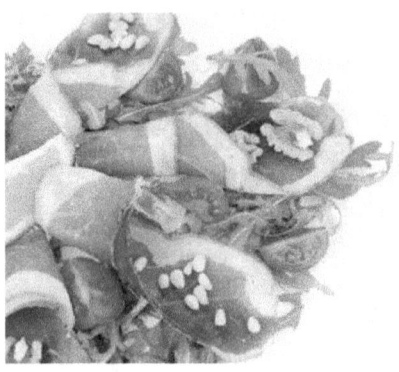

SERVES: 4

INGREDIENTS:

- 2 cups quinces, peeled and core removed, quartered
- 2 to 3 tablespoons of local honey
- Zest of 1/2 lemon, sliced into strips
- 4 cups baby arugula
- ½ cup Serrano ham or prosciutto ham, thinly sliced
- 2 Tbs. extra-virgin olive oil

- Kosher salt, to taste
- Black pepper, freshly ground to taste
- ¼ cup almonds, toasted and chopped
- ¼ cup firm Manchego or Asiago, or other mild-flavored cheeses, shaved
- 4 balsamic vinegar, preferably aged 12 to 25 years

DIRECTIONS:

1. Place the quartered quinces, organic zest of lemon and 3 tablespoons of local honey in a pan. Pour water to cover the quinces with 1 inch. Apply medium-high heat, bring to a boil and then cover with lid. Reduce to low heat and simmer for about 40 to 45 minutes. The quinces are ready when it is soft and tender. Remove from heat, set aside to cool.

2. Toss in arugula, the ham, in a mixing bowl and stir in the oil. Adjust seasoning with salt and ground black pepper. Portion the salad among serving plates. Add the quinces over the salad plates. Top off with shaved Manchego cheese and chopped almonds, drizzle salad with balsamic vinegar. Serve.

Farro Salad with Marinated Artichokes, Watercress, and Feta

Farro is a nutty, chewy grain once it's cooked, that was used by the ancient Romans.

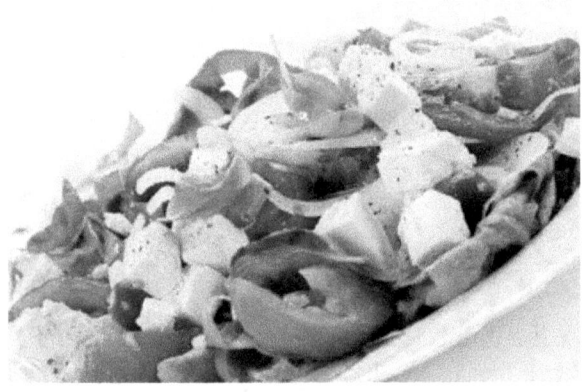

SERVES: 4

INGREDIENTS:

FOR THE ARTICHOKES:

- 2 tablespoons fresh oregano
- 1 1/2 cups extra-virgin olive oil, or as needed
- 1/2 cup white wine vinegar
- ½ cup fresh parsley

- ¼ cup fresh thyme
- 2 garlic cloves, peeled and crushed
- salt
- 4 artichokes, trimmed, and quartered

FOR THE SALAD:

- salt
- 1 cup farro
- 1 cup Feta cheese or goat's cheese
- 2 medium scallions, cut into bias
- ½ cup watercress, trimmed and chopped
- 2 teaspoons red wine vinegar
- Freshly cracked black pepper

DIRECTIONS:

1. Add 1 cup water, garlic, salt, vinegar in a pot over high heat and bring to a boil. Add the artichokes and cook until tender, or for about 10 minutes. Remove artichokes from pot and drain, pat dry with paper towels. Transfer in a bowl and add in the garlic, parsley, thyme,

oregano and pour over the oil. Set aside and let it sit for about 1 hour.

2. Drain the artichokes and reserve ¼ cup of oil, discard garlic and herbs. Return artichokes and reserved oil in the bowl.

3. In a pan with salted boiling water, add and cook the faro for about 20 to 25 minutes. Drain and place on a baking sheet to cool.

4. Mix in cooked farro in the bowl with artichokes and oil. Let it rest for about 10 minutes to infuse the flavors. Mix in watercress and vinegar, season with salt and pepper to taste. Serve.

Grilled Eggplant Salad with Feta, Pine Nuts & Garlicky Yogurt Dressing

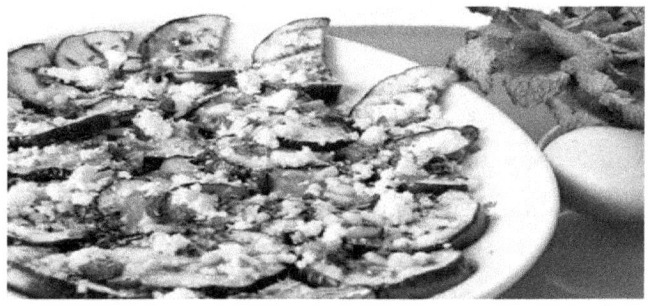

SERVES: 4

INGREDIENTS:

- 2 heads of romaine lettuce, leaves separated
- 1 large eggplant, halved and sliced
- 4 tablespoons extra-virgin olive oil
- ½ cup Greek yogurt
- ½ organic lemon, juiced
- 2 cloves of garlic, mashed into paste
- A pinch of ground cumin
- ½ cup fresh flat-leaf parsley leaves, minced
- ½ cup Feta cheese or goat's cheese, crumbled
- ¼ cup pine nuts, toasted

DIRECTIONS:

1. Place lettuce leaves in a bowl and cover with paper towels, chill.
2. Preheat gas grill with high heat, brush eggplant with 2 tablespoons of oil and season with salt and pepper. Reduce gas grill to low heat and grill the eggplant for about 3 minutes on each side. Flip to cook the other side, cook for 3 minutes. Remove from grill and transfer to a plate.
3. Remove lettuce from the chiller and portion into individual serving plates, top with grilled eggplant, feta and nuts then drizzle with dressing on top.

Tomato Salad with Feta, Olives & Mint

Similar to a traditional Greek salad, but the addition of mint and lemon freshens and lightens it.

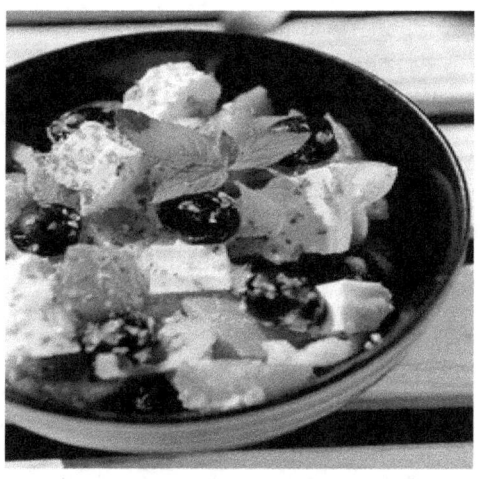

SERVES: 6

INGREDIENTS:

- 1 cup Feta cheese, crumbled
- 1/4 cup fresh mint, chopped
- 4 ripe red tomatoes, sliced into thin rounds
- Kosher salt

- 2 medium cucumber, peeled and seeded, diced
- 1 cup cherry tomatoes, halved
- 1/2 cup Kalamata olives, pitted and halved
- 4 tablespoons extra virgin olive oil
- ½ tablespoon grated organic lemon zest
- 1 tablespoon fresh organic lemon juice
- Freshly cracked black pepper

DIRECTIONS:

1. In a mixing bowl, combine cheese and mint and set aside.
2. Sprinkle with salt and pepper over the tomato slices and arrange them on a serving platter. Add the cucumbers and olives on top and chill.
3. Whisk together the oil, lemon juice and zest, salt and pepper in a bowl. Drizzle mixture over the salad and top with cheese. Serve immediately.

Conclusion

For us, it's so inspiring that eating means sharing. The coming together of friends and family to share a meal is one of the most powerful and intimate forms of communication that there is. Mealtimes should always be special occasions, richly blessed with togetherness, light-hearted conversation, and wonderful health-giving ingredients. Food for family and friends is less about spending hours in the kitchen, and more about simply opening the door to those you love and offering to share what you have.

Mediterranean principles teach us that the best meals are often the simplest, provided they are prepared with respect for good ingredients and plenty of care. So you may only have a simple salad and a loaf of crusty bread, but when offered with generosity and a spirit of hospitality, they become a feast fit for royalty.
We trust that these recipes will become well-used and well-loved in your household, and that you will have as much fun making them as we have had putting them together.

www.ingramcontent.com/pod-product-compliance
Lightning Source LLC
LaVergne TN
LVHW010315070526
838199LV00065B/5571